Holistic Medicine
Beyond the Physical

Dr Carol Head

National Library of Australia Cataloguing-in-Publication entry (pbk)

Creator: Head, Carol A. author.

Title: Holistic medicine : beyond the physical / Carol Head.

ISBN: 9780994233509 (paperback)

ISBN: 9780994233516 (ebook)

Subjects: Holistic medicine.

                 Mind and body.

                 Spiritual care (Medical care)

                 Intuition.

Dewey Number: 615.8528

Book Cover Layout: Laila Savolainen (Pickawoowoo Publishing Group)

Publishing Consultants - Pickawoowoo Publishing Group

Dr Carol Head

Web: www.drcarolhead.com.au

Email: drcarolhead@gmail.com

In Memory of Angela Leehane

One doesn't discover new lands without consenting to lose sight of the shore

Andre Gide

Table of Contents

INTRODUCTION

This book is about a different way of viewing the world. It is not about a set of rules on how to live your life. It is not about following a number of steps to reach a goal. It is about viewing life as an unfolding process and about learning how we might better become part of that process, so that instead of resisting the process of life we learn how to live it.

This is not easy because we keep teaching our children to view the world in a particular way. We learn a particular view of the world from our parents and the society in which we live. But what if our problems as a species arise from the way we view the world? What if our view of the world causes much of our suffering?

When I was young, I was taught that the world worked in a certain way. I was taught that if I logically planned my life and worked hard then I would be happy. I was given a list of rules to live my life by. Unfortunately someone gave me the wrong instruction manual.

My society and my culture gave me a set of rules to live by and told me over and over again that if I just followed the rules and did what I was meant to do I would be happy. Whenever life seemed to go wrong, I assumed that I wasn't following the rules properly, that somehow I had failed, that I wasn't doing well enough.

This instruction manual isn't written down. It's passed down from generation to generation. The rules are taught at school and in the workplace and in the media.

It only took me about forty years to realise that the problem wasn't me, it was the instruction manual and the set of rules that my culture had taught me. I could write chapters on the problems with our society's instruction manual but in a way that is useless. We all know the problems that occur when we use the wrong manual – it doesn't work, we get confused, lost, frustrated, depressed, and our life feels wrong. We feel that we don't fit, we don't belong. Our lives are spent desperately searching for something. Only we don't know that what we are searching for is the right instruction manual because we don't realise that we have the wrong one.

At the age of forty-two, I began the conscious search for a better instruction manual. I cast aside my 'how to live in Western patriarchal society as a female doctor and mother' and picked up the 'how to live in Western society as a spiritual being' manual. Thinking they were wrong, I put aside my old set of rules and took up a new set, thinking they were right. Of course, they weren't. I moved closer to what felt like a fit but still at times I felt confused and frustrated. Mostly, I thought I just couldn't do the rules right, when all along I still didn't have the right manual or the right rules.

So at the age of forty-five, I began to write my own. It began as a book about the spiritual side of life that Western society ignores, but it has evolved into a very different book. Interestingly, before I could even begin to grasp what it was about I had called it Holistic Medicine. I knew the topic, I just didn't know all the content. I learnt about the content of this book through the process and flow of my life. The lessons I learnt as I lived my life were the lessons I needed to learn in order to be able to write this book. The latest lesson has been the most difficult. That is the lesson on how to finish the book.

That lesson is about my being willing to have a book that is not perfect, that does not have the answer that will fix everyone's problems. The lesson I had to learn was that my role as doctor/ teacher/healer is as much about healing myself and learning about myself as it is about helping others to learn and heal. I had to unlearn my first rule of medicine, which has always been to try to fix the problem.

This book is not about fixing problems. It is about shining light onto problems. It is about seeing problems for what they really are. It is about examining our lives for clues about how we might live happier and healthier.

This book is my attempt to put together an instruction manual for living a whole life. It is not perfect and it is not truth. There will be parts of it that will need changing as time goes on. But it is a start.

I began this book over ten years ago. It had been ideas swirling around in my head for many years but I couldn't find the time to begin it. Then one of my best friends died quite suddenly. Angela was younger than I was and she lived down the road. She had three children similar in age to mine and our daughters were best friends. At that stage, I had been separated for three years and Angela and her family were a great support to my children and me. She was like a sister to me and our relationship was completely uncomplicated. On 15 August 2004, Angela collapsed behind the shed on her property. Her husband, Bill, tried to revive her, and the ambulance came and took her to hospital, but there was nothing anyone could do. At the age of thirty-seven, Angela was dead, of causes unknown.

This event had a profound effect on me. I realised a number of things. I realised that Angela's presence was still around at times – that something lives on after we physically die. I realised that any one of us could die at any moment and that I shouldn't waste my time doing things that weren't important to me. I realised that no matter how much I talked about writing a book, it wouldn't happen unless I actually did it. So I quit my job and started to write.

Why Angela died will always be a mystery to me but the meaning I have found in her death led me to write this book – so it is that I dedicate this book to her.

This book is about my version of holistic medicine, which I will define as the art and science of helping people learn how to heal themselves.

There are a number of assumptions I make about holistic medicine. The first is that holistic medicine is about learning how to heal. Healing is not something that someone does to you but something you do to yourself. Holistic medicine teaches people how to heal themselves. It is not about teaching people how to heal themselves but about teaching people to learn how to heal. We have forgotten that we can all heal ourselves. The healing comes about when we allow ourselves to be whole people. Of course our bodies heal naturally much of the time, so holistic medicine is also about promoting this natural healing power we already have.

The second assumption is that everyone is unique and the only person who can learn how to heal you is you. We are all different and what we need to learn in this life is different. I do not know the answers to your problems but I can help you learn how to find them. The responsibility for your own healing lies with you, the responsibility for wholeness lies with you.

The third assumption is that we are all whole people but that we have forgotten how to live as whole people. We have forgotten about some of our parts and we have forgotten that life is a process; that it goes in cycles and spirals and vortices. The whole is made up of content – the parts, and process – the movement of life. But we cannot dissect the whole to find all our answers. We find most of our answers to our deepest healing by living the whole thing – living our life. Living our life – not someone else's.

There is no definitive Western model of holistic medicine, so this is my attempt to write about one. Of course, it won't be definitive because it is just my version.

I have divided the book into four parts. The first attempts to define a holistic model of the human system. I look at the content of the system and the processes that the system operates under.

The second part looks in greater detail at the parts of the system and the processes.

The third part outlines some of the theory behind holism and the differences between our current world view and a holistic world view.

The fourth part looks at how we can consciously pay attention to our physical and spiritual aspects and learn through the process of our lives more about who we really are and what we need as individuals to be whole people. This is how we heal ourselves.

I make no claims that this book or my view of the world is any more correct than anyone else's. What I believe is that if we pay attention to our lives in a conscious way, we can find our own path to healing and wholeness. The models and framework that I put forward are just models. This is a way of looking at something that is enormously complex (the human system) in a simpler way so that we can be more aware of why we get sick and why we get stuck in our problems. Like all models and theories, use only the parts that are useful to you as an individual. There is no such thing as one right answer. The meaning of life is found as we live our own life.

PART ONE

THE HUMAN SYSTEM

The soul is its own source of unfolding

Heraclitus

ONE - WHO AM I?

The human system is so immensely complex that to simplify it into an understandable model is impossible. Nevertheless, I am going to try. I will begin with the simplest ideas and gradually enlarge them and build on the basics. However, it is important to understand that the more you think about it the more confused you can sometimes become. So do not think too much, do not try to grasp the concepts too hard or they will slip away. Much of what we need to understand about ourselves we understand through experiencing it.

The simplest concept to begin with is that we are like the point zero symbol.

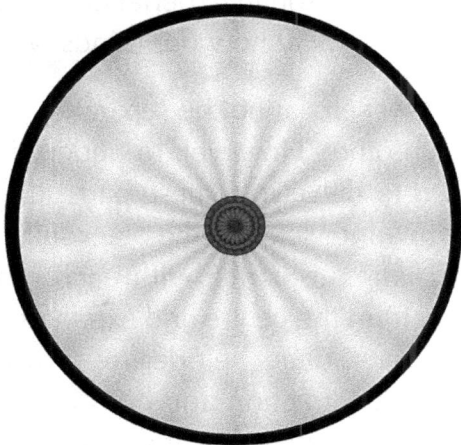

We are made up of two basic parts. The inner self – the point, and the outer self – the circle (zero).

The inner self, the point, is our essential nature, our soul. This is the part of us that at its very essence is unchanging and that makes us a unique individual. This deep self is also connected to everything else in ways we don't fully understand. The connection is to other people but also to the whole system. Some people consider this part of our self to be our spiritual self. Others might call it the observing self.

The circle is, in simple terms, our outer persona, the face we show the world. It is also the connections we have with other people and things in the physical world. The circle also signifies the process of life that we continually undergo, the cycles of life that make it so hard to pin any of this down, because it is always changing form; life is always moving.

As humans we understand things in two main ways. We understand something by first breaking it down into its parts (reductionism) and then gaining an understanding of the whole thing. Or we accept or know that something is whole and we understand how it works through experiencing it. I will discuss this concept further when I look at how our minds work.

Inner self and outer self cannot be separated in real life because they are part of each other. However, to understand how we work as humans we need to delve into these parts. It is as if our whole self is made up of the inner self and the outer self but the two selves are involved in an intricate dance with each other. Outer self is always pulling away from the centre and expanding and inner self is always trying to contract. Outer self desires growth and expansion and inner self desires contraction and consolidation.[1] We are like a plant growing towards the sun but if we don't also grow into the earth, we will topple over.

---

1   Or we could look at it from a different direction and say that inner self desires expansion and outer self desires contraction – it is the same thing.

Part of us is always looking for growth opportunities, changing in response to the external environment, and part of us is looking for safety and stability. This is like yin and yang. Yang is light, and expansive; yin is dark and contracting. We are made up of both these parts. Because we have these two parts, we sometimes feel as if we are being pulled in two directions.

Plants don't look at it like that. Plants just live – they send parts of themselves up into the light, to grow and expand, and they send other parts deep into the earth, also to grow and expand but invisibly. Which part is the real plant?

Humans, unlike other species, have consciousness. We are conscious that we are, that we exist. The other side of this is that we are also partly unconscious. So while we believe we have control over our lives and over ourselves, this is only partly true. Our unconscious is also partly in charge, but it works in the dark, anchoring us, stopping us from toppling over. We don't understand this side of ourselves and it scares the hell out of us. We fear this part of ourselves because we don't understand it.

This unconscious earthing of the human system underpins the theory of holistic medicine. Holistic medicine is about helping people learn how to heal themselves. The unconscious processes that happen to us, that we believe are caused by external factors, are actually trying to bring about our healing. Healing is about becoming whole. We become whole (in the simplest of terms) when we balance the needs of our inner and outer selves. We balance the expansion and the contraction. We balance the growth and the consolidation. We grow towards the light and into the earth. We are pulled by a physical desire to be separate and individual, and a spiritual desire to be one with everything else.

Our balance is best served by allowing the expansion and contraction to occur naturally. It is like breathing in and out. But we have all forgotten how to do this naturally. Western society teaches us how to expand but not how to contract. We breathe in and in and in and then we can't get the air out. We are full of good ideas and brilliant plans but we run ourselves into the ground because we have forgotten how to ground ourselves in the earth.

The human system is very similar to the sphere that is the planet earth. Take a look at the front cover and pay attention to what the earth looks like from space.

One half is light and one half is dark. This is what we are like. We are half light and half dark.

Most Western culture has classified the light and dark as opposing forces. It has divided life into a series of lines. In this way, Western society classifies everything – good and bad, right and wrong, god and devil, heaven and earth.

Much of Eastern culture in contrast (and remember this is contrast for the sake of contrast) takes the view that life on earth is not real, that our physical life is an illusion of the spirit. This view sees humans as spiritual beings whose only job is to reach enlightenment, and the way to enlightenment is to follow the light. It seeks to transcend the physical and become pure spirit.

The West aligns itself with the physical dimensions; the physical body and logical thinking. The East aligns itself with the spiritual dimensions; feelings and intuition.

Who is right?

Neither and both.

Neither is absolutely right and both are partially right.

Take another look at the earth.

Both Eastern and Western traditions seek to shed light on the dark side. In the west, we do this by adding more light. We shine our light on everything trying to find greater understanding. Similarly, in the east the task is enlightenment; bringing our conscious awareness to every part of our lives. So our whole lives become a struggle.

The earth does not need to be all light. In fact, if it were it would die, as it would if it were all dark. But we humans have convinced ourselves that dark is bad and light is good so we are always seeking more light.

The earth as a system has only one task. To stay alive. To do this it must try to stay in balance. As long as it can stay in balance it can stay alive. If it falls out of balance it will die. Of course, dying is not all that bad because it is part of the great cycle of life but for each person on earth, for each animal, for each plant, the whole aim of being here is to live. This may be self-evident but it seems we have forgotten it.

Living is not good enough any more. We think we have to live a certain way. Well, this model of holistic medicine says differently. All we have to do is live our life.

We are here to live.

We are here to live our cycle. The cycle is birth, life, death, birth, life, death. And no matter whether we believe this or not, this is the cycle. We can rage against this and convince ourselves that we do not have to die or that we do not have to live, but the reality of this world is that we will all die. This is part of the nature of the world we live in. We do not know what is beyond the three physical dimensions and we will not know until we die. But that is not the point of life. The point of life is to live so we can know and experience what life is all about.

This is the meaning of life – to live. To enter into the process of our very own life and see where it goes. To embrace our whole self and use our parts in the way they were intended.

Who am I?

I am human.

To be human is to embrace the whole self – the dark and the light, the physical and the spiritual, the conscious and the unconscious, the expansion and the contraction.

The inner and the outer self (dark and light, physical and spiritual, conscious and unconscious) are connected to each other. They are connected in two ways, and again we consider the earth.

Picture the earth again – it is half light, half dark. The light half is the conscious half. On this side, people are awake and active. The sun is fuelling physical growth and helping maintain the balance, but there are shadows where the sun does not reach. The dark half is the unconscious half. Here, people are asleep and refuelling themselves. The moon and stars are providing some light so it is never completely dark. Each half is mostly either light or dark with some of its opposite. This is the mix; this is the content of life.

Now picture the earth turning and see the edge of light taking over the dark. On the other side of the earth we would see the edge of dark taking over the light. As light recedes, dark expands, as dark recedes, light expands. This is part of the dance; this is the process of life.

Now picture the earth stopping still. Imagine what happens when the earth stops. Pretty soon – nothing. Life is as much about the movement and process as it is about the content and the parts. Process is the movement of our lives that occurs over time. There are no constants in life, it is always moving, always in process.

The Taoist symbol of yin and yang illustrates these concepts as well.

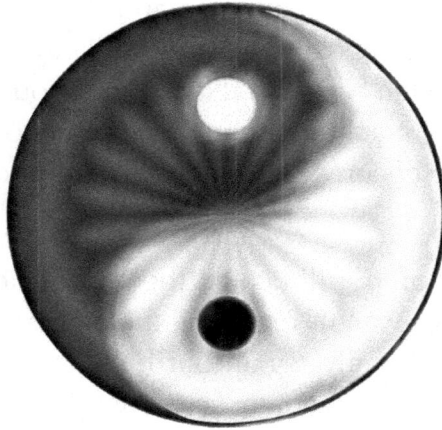

Yang is the light and yin is the dark. Some call yang physical and yin spiritual but for each of us this is different. For some of us our yang is more physical and for some it is more spiritual. This is dependent upon our individual makeup. For the moment, let's just look at yang as light and yin as dark.

In yang there is a small bit of yin, and in yin there is also some yang. Each of us is made up of our unique mix of light and dark. The mix is who you are.

The curved line symbolises the dance between yin and yang; as yang expands yin contracts and as yin expands yang contracts. Life is one continual dance between the yin and the yang, between expansion and contraction. We dance between the needs of our physical self and those of our spiritual self. The dance is also who we are.

We are the mix and we are the dance. Our mix and our dance are always changing in response to the world around us and the world around us is changing in response to us.

When we overbalance in either direction – too much expansion and growth or too much contraction and stability – life has to flow in the other direction. Because we are not always consciously aware of this process, it often happens at an unconscious level. In this way, if we expand or contract too much then our unconscious pushes us the other way. We become sick – mentally, physically, emotionally, or spiritually.

At the basis of all our ill health, then, is this idea of imbalance. Illness is the body's way of regaining the balance. We can go with this process and naturally regain our balance, or we can become conscious of the process and consciously bring ourselves back into balance.

Of course this is an oversimplification but it helps to illustrate the concept of holistic medicine. Holistic medicine aims to help people learn how to regain their balance and live whole.

As we find our balance, which is half spiritual and half physical (just like the earth), we feel perfect and at peace and full of love. Occasionally we attain this at certain times and we know that this is who we really are. When we enter this timeless spaceless zone, we know that we are exactly as we should be, that we are perfect. This is what we are searching for and when we find it we know. Most of us have felt like this at some moment in our lives. Perfect. The moment is perfect just as it is.

But then the music changes and we go out of balance and so the dance is on again. But what we realise at some of those perfect moments is that we have much to learn about how to stay in better balance.

This is our holy grail. Perfect balance, perfect harmony, when our physical body and our mind are totally in harmony with our spiritual body and mind and our whole self fits into its place in the universe.

The conflict we all feel is because we are not conscious of how we work. We don't realise that we have a continuous conflict between the perceived needs of our two halves. We have a spiritual need to achieve oneness with everything else, unity with all that is. But our physical side needs separation, to be a unique and separate being. So there is a continuous conflict between what we perceive are our physical and spiritual needs.

When we examine it, we might conclude differently. Imagine we are all individual drops of water in the giant ocean of life. We know we are part of a greater whole but we know we are different from the other drops because we move up against them and make waves and ripples.

If we are able to attain perfect balance between our two halves and everything and everyone else is able to attain perfect balance, then the ripples between us all stop. We are perfectly balanced and not sending out ripples, everyone else is perfectly balanced and not sending out ripples. Suddenly the sea is still, there are no ripples, no waves, no dance, no signs of life, nothing. We are in a void.

How do we know we are alive in a void?

Only by the dancing.

We can theorise about what is after this life or before it, what exists in other dimensions, but all that does is take our attention away from the dance.

We have two major fears – total obliteration or total union with all that is. The only way that I can be me is to avoid both these scenarios and ultimately both these fears are the same thing. Either way I cease to exist.

Western society and its set of rules forgot to tell me all of this. It had me convinced I was mainly a physical being and it had me convinced that life followed a straight line and that I was separate from everyone else.

This book begins with three different assumptions.

We are half physical and half spiritual and both halves are equally important.

Life follows a process and the process is more complex than a straight line, it is like a dance.

We are all dancing together.

Further to this I believe that no particular mix of physical and spiritual characteristics is any better than any other mix. We all dance differently but no-one's dance is any better than anyone else's. What we each seek is to understand our own mix and to learn how to follow the dance better. We seek to discover the parts of ourselves that we have forgotten, and we seek to learn how to live the process of life more smoothly, and we do this with everyone else.

This is at the heart of every person's individual quest; this is how we find the meaning in our lives. The meaning is actually very simple – we are here to be our self. Our unique individual self. We are here to bring our uniqueness into the physical reality of this world. Shine our light. Be authentic. Follow our path.

We are not here to be someone else.

We are here to be ourselves.

Yet this is no easy task because we are brought up in our society to believe we should be something other than who we are. We learn many ways to hide who we really are. Some of us learn how to hide who we really are even from ourselves, so it takes us many years to realise that who we seem to be is not who we really are. It is no wonder that most of us are sick, anxious and depressed. We are severely out of balance. We are trying to be someone we are not.

This person that we all try to be is some idealised version of our self. This idealised version arises from all the influences that we have had in our childhood, and in our society it is inevitable. Maybe this is part of some grand scheme. To me it doesn't matter. My aim is to help people live whole. This wholeness in the simplest terms means being the person you are meant to be. Being yourself. Part of being yourself is being involved in the dance of life with everyone else. We do not exist in isolation and this is the tricky part of the dance. We must find our place in the giant web of life (the dance). We appear to have a conflict between wanting separation and wanting connectedness but this is just because we have not found our place in the web – we are trying to be someone we are not.

Yin and Yang

In Western society we have no words that directly translate yin and yang. These words describe a perspective and their definition is not simple. I am going to use these words throughout the book so I will attempt to give the reader some idea of their meaning.

Yin and yang are used extensively in Chinese medicine and their meaning encompasses the difference between Western and Eastern world views.

Chinese view the universe as constantly changing, it has an essential movement that doesn't result from any one cause but is the result of a cyclical pattern.

In the West, we always seek to find a cause for events and ultimately, it seems, a creator of all events. Eastern metaphysics is concerned not with causative agents but with patterns, cycles and relationships.[2] Yin and yang are part of the explanation of how the patterns and cycles occur and how everything relates to everything else.

Yin and yang are not things but rather they explain the continuous process of natural change. So they describe qualities of things.

Everything can be described by its yin and yang qualities and everything has both qualities. A human being is both yin and yang. The earth is yin and yang. The yin and yang qualities are descriptors that apply in relation to something else, both within and without the system. So a man might be yang in comparison to a woman but might be yin in relationship to another man (although these are not constants, so sometimes a man will be yin in relationship to a woman.)

Yang and yin aspects can also be divided ad infinitum so that in yang, there is always some yin and in yin, there is always some yang. The two aspects are always flowing from one state to another so that yin gives way to yang and yang gives way to yin. They are not fixed things; they signify the movement of the cosmos.

---

2   Something that the New physics is also now concerned with – see part 3, chapter 2.

Yang qualities are masculine while yin qualities are feminine. Yang is assertive and outgoing, yin is receptive and introspective. These qualities both oppose and balance each other. They set the limits of the natural cycle. Once yang is maximum it must give way to yin, and vice-versa. Yang is the breath in and yin the breath out. Yin is the filling of the heart with blood and yang the contraction of the heart and expulsion of blood. Life is the intricate dance between these two qualities.

Two -
The five elements

M y holistic model of the human system moves beyond its most basic theme – light and dark, physical and spiritual, to a more complex model. The human system can be divided into four basic elements or aspects. Each element is very complex and as we come to understand these elements, we come to understand ourselves better.

The elements are air, fire, water, and earth. If you like to divide the light and dark halves into two again, then the light (or yang) half is fire and air and the dark (or yin) half is water and earth. I will give

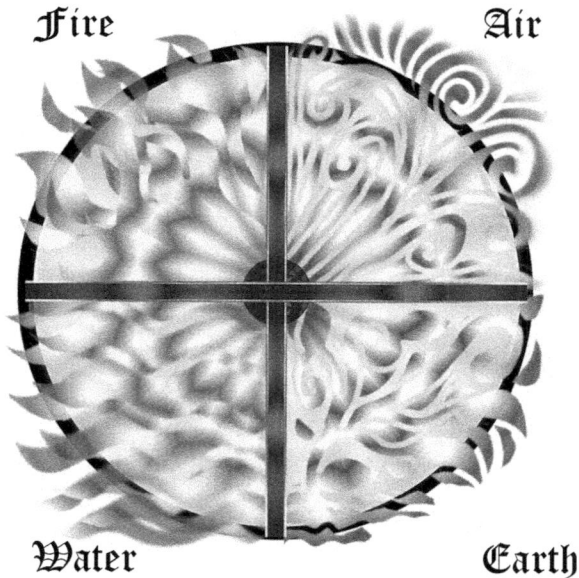

Fire   Air

Water   Earth

a brief description of each element in this chapter, and later go on to describe them in more detail.

Air – Mind

Air is the element of thought. This is the human mind and it is a very complex thing. So I am going to divide it first into two parts, which correspond to the two sides of the brain.[3] This is a somewhat simplistic view of the brain, but it helps us to understand it better than if we believe the brain just thinks in one way.

The brain is divided into two hemispheres, imaginatively called the right hemisphere and the left hemisphere. These two sides of the brain think in two different ways.

The left side of the brain thinks in logical, rational ways. This is what some people call our intellect. It breaks problems down into parts (called reductionism) and seeks to solve problems by examining the parts. It thinks in black and white terms, right and wrong, good and bad (called dualism). Left-brain thinking is called rational thinking (this is also known as linear thinking).

The right side of the brain thinks intuitively, in wholes, in systems (called holism). It thinks creatively, laterally, imaginatively. Right-brain thinking is called intuitive thinking (also known as non-linear thinking) and it is not logical.

The left side thinks mainly in words and numbers, the right mainly in pictures and patterns and symbols. So language is primarily a left-brain concept while pictures and symbols are right brain territory.

---

3   You can begin to see that to understand the whole in this model (the human system) we first have to divide it into smaller and smaller parts. This is only a model. The parts are not really separate things, they only exist as part of the system.

Our thinking appears to be done by our left brain; we think in words, we have a train of thought expressed in words and sentences. These thoughts lead onto other thoughts in a linear fashion and we reach a conclusion. Or the thoughts go round in circles and we get confused. This is all left-brain thinking (of course this is an oversimplification but we need to simplify for the left brain to understand).

Our right brain thinks in a different way. The right brain seems to come up with an answer suddenly. It doesn't use the left brain's linear processing to find the answer methodically and logically. Rather, it synthesises all the information in a different way and seems to then suddenly know the answer to a problem, or it suddenly grasps an issue and understands it. As the right brain doesn't use words and sentences to think, we often assume it is silent, but it just uses a different process to the left brain.

Neither hemisphere can think in isolation; they are joined primarily by a structure called the corpus callosum, a network of connections that link both hemispheres. The distinction between the two sides is partly academic but it helps us understand the two different processes that occur in our brains. Where they occur anatomically isn't very important for most of us.

Conventional scientific thought uses both sides of the brain but believes that the left side is superior. Science and medicine believe that reductionism and dualism are a superior way of thinking and working out problems compared to holism. They believe truth is to be found in logic and rational analysis.[4]

As individuals and as a society (which includes medicine), what is needed is not a greater reliance on either side of the brain but the

4   Of course the progressive branches of science – notably physics – believe that holism is the new direction of science, but the biological sciences are still stuck in the old scientific ways. I will explore this further in Part three – Holistic Theory.

ability to use both sides together and also to use either side in the way it works best.

The left side works best for analysing and logically sorting out problems, by reducing the problem into parts and analysing the parts. The left brain can't conceptualise the whole thing except by looking at the parts.

The right side works best when looking at the whole picture, establishing patterns, and intuitive thinking and creativity. The right brain can't understand how the parts fit together except by looking at the whole.

Most of us in Western society are out of balance (too left brained) and the reason for this is because it is what we have learnt. We have learnt, in the past few centuries, to use our logical rational brain over our intuitive non-rational brain.

Earth and water – Body

As well as dividing the mind into two parts we can divide the body into two – the physical body (earth) and the feeling body (water).

Our physical body is fairly obvious, although many of us try to deny that we have a body that actually needs looking after. We try to use the power of our logical mind to control our body, to make it do what we want. In our culture, we are taught to disregard the messages from our body. We run marathons and compete in sports that stress our bodies and then wonder why our bodies let us down. We feed our bodies a diet of junk (both physical and emotional) and then wonder why they don't work well.

Not only are we taught to disregard our physical bodies, we are also taught to disregard our emotional bodies. We learn early on that some emotions are just not okay – for me it was anger and frustration and hate. I learnt that I should always be happy and caring and love everyone. I learnt the Western idea of 'good' and I tried to follow this. That meant I had to suppress any emotion that was not perceived by society as 'good'.

Fire

At its simplest, fire is the part of us that drives us to grow and create. It is the passion that burns, the creative flame that leads us to great works of art or scientific discoveries. It is the part of us that seeks to grow and expand. Fire is our closest link to the spiritual world. Our intuitive abilities stem from fire, but we experience them through our other elements. Like all our elements, fire has two sides and its potential for destruction is greater than the other elements.

So here we have the concept of four elements – fire, air, water, and earth. Western society values fire and has a heavy reliance on left brain over right brain (unbalanced air). It devalues the physical and emotional bodies (earth and water). So most of us are unbalanced, or living in a society that is unbalanced. Yet despite this, the human system has the uncanny ability to find its own balance and to continue living and growing.

Before we look at how the human system does this, let's just take a step back and look at how we come to know that we are an individual.

Ego

Our ego develops during our childhood in order for us to separate from our parents. Our ego is essential for our physical existence because it provides us with our individuality – our firm conviction that we are a separate individual. It gives us a sense of having our own physical identity, which we believe is quite separate from every other person. This is only half the truth because we are also connected to every other person, however our physical presence is the symbol of our individuality.

The ego provides us with our identity and we come to believe that who we think we are is who we really are. Prior to our being able to think in our native language (as infants), there is no doubt we still existed – but we were largely unaware that we existed because we didn't have a language to think in. So we develop this idea of ourselves as being who we 'think' we are.

We all 'think' using the left side of our brain. The left side of the brain is where we have the thoughts that are made up of words and sentences and some images. We think using our left brain in what is called 'linear thinking'. One thought leads to another and another. This is our logic, our rational thinking, and this is the part of the brain that we typically believe is who we are. This part of our brain rules our conscious awareness because this is what we have been taught in Western society. We have been taught to use our left brain and to rely on it for solving our problems.

We are, however, more complex than this, it is just that we are not consciously aware of all our aspects or parts. Some of our parts are below our conscious awareness (subconscious or unconscious).

Our ego, from which we derive our sense of self in the physical world, takes on various sets of belief systems. These belief systems are ideas we have about how the world works and where we fit into it. They are not truth but we often believe they are truth. We rarely question our own belief systems.

Our belief system comes about largely through external influences. What our parents, friends, families, teachers, churches, governments, and the rest of society tell us influences what we believe to be true.

As children and adolescents, we take a lot of notice of these external messages about how the world works and who we are. Sometimes as adults, we continue to let our lives be ruled by a belief system that is dictated by other people. Our ego (the ideas we have about who we are) helps maintain the illusion that what we believe is actually truth. We believe what we learn to believe and we think our beliefs are truth.

Ego is like a bridge between the physical world and the spiritual world. This consciously aware part of our whole self is what we need to live in a physical world. The physical world is limited – three dimensions of space and one of time – but the spiritual world (I believe) is unlimited. To live in a limited world with unlimited consciousness would be impossible, so we have the protection of ego. Ego lets certain traffic onto the bridge of awareness. It lets traffic on that it believes we can cope with and it closes the bridge to traffic that it believes will harm us.

Ego acts as a gatekeeper – it filters information from the physical world and information from the spiritual world and delivers what it believes is useful to our conscious awareness.

When we are egocentric, we are mostly focused on the traffic coming from our external world. We are living from a perspective that sees us as totally separate from the rest of the system. We focus on the traffic from the material world and don't pay enough attention to the traffic coming the other way. We often end up with confusion. As we become more aware, we begin to pay attention to the traffic coming from our inner self, our soul, our internal world, the spiritual dimensions. We keep paying attention to the external traffic but now we are conscious that both external and internal realities exist.

(Some people might view external as being the spiritual dimension and internal as being the physical. That's fine. What is important is that we pay both halves attention.)

The soul or inner reality is always sending messages to the conscious part of ourselves – the bridge as it were – but we have been taught to mistrust these messages. We believe that we should pay more attention to the external world. So then the soul, of necessity, creates the experience we need to make us start to question our beliefs. This is the process of life, and it opens us up to the parts of ourselves that we haven't been paying enough attention to. We become more conscious of how we limit our own growth by limiting our beliefs about what is possible. We close our minds and we shut the bridge.

The bridge works best when it is open both ways, when traffic can flow. We shut it when we don't listen to our spiritual self just as surely as when we don't listen to our physical self. Our ego self expands as it opens the bridge between outer and inner worlds.

Part of the trouble as I see it is that Western society has given control of ego to the logical mind. Remember this is a metaphor – it won't necessarily make logical sense. I am trying to get this information into your ego, your conscious awareness, and so I have to use terms that it understands or it will just filter out what I am saying. When we give control of the ego to our logical mind, we filter out everything that isn't logical. So we filter out the two main channels that give us information from our spiritual self – our feelings and our intuition.

Soul – Inner Self

Imagine your soul, or inner self, as the spiritual essence of who you are. Most of us will have trouble imagining this because we see ourselves as our thinking brain. We have come to believe that the voice in our head is us. The voice in our head is part of us but it is only our ego, it is not the whole of us and it is not who we really are. Imagine that if there is a part of you that is eternal, what that part would be like.

Imagine then that your soul has been hidden for many years under the accumulated stuff of your life – the job, the hobbies, the relationships, the roles you have taken on, the material stuff you own, the beliefs that you hold in your conscious mind, the things you think you should do, and the ways you think you should act and behave.

Imagine that your inner self is not happy with this state of affairs, that it is sick of being ignored. What could it do?

I imagine it has a number of choices but because we are physical beings, its choices are limited by the physical reality we live in. It has to reach our conscious awareness but to do this it has to get past our ego. Ego, our conscious awareness, protects us from too much information. It protects us from all the stuff in our unconscious mind that we are not able to deal with at this moment. We cannot deal with being conscious of too much information so all information that wants access to our conscious awareness has to go through ego.[5]

So let's imagine a bridge between our physical self and our spiritual self, where ego sits on the bridge protecting our sense of individuality. Ego assesses all the information coming to it from our external physical world and from the internal spiritual world. It decides what to take most notice of at any one time. Because we are

---

5   Remember this is a metaphor or model, not truth, but just a way to view ourselves so that we might understand ourselves better. The truth is obviously more complex than this.

brought up in a Western culture, our ego is a Western ego and it pays most attention to the logical rational information and the left brain.

Ego sits on the bridge and along comes some information from our inner self.

'Hello ego,' it might say, 'I am the inner self, let me into your awareness.' (Remember this isn't logical – if you try to make it fit into a logical framework you will drive yourself crazy.)

Ego checks with logical mind, who most likely says something like, 'Ego you're going crazy there isn't anything there. Listen to me you idiot, I am in control, there is no such thing as inner self or soul. Someone is playing a trick on you.'

So inner self has to use the channels open to it. It can't just jump into our awareness fully formed, it has to creep in bit by bit. The way it does this is through the four elements.

Inner self might try to reach our consciousness through feelings. In my experience this will often manifest initially as a feeling of sadness or loss, or anxiety and depression. Most of us ignore these feelings, try to rationalise them away.

'Why should I feel like this? I have a great family, a good job, and good friends,' the left brain rationalises.

But still we feel slightly unbalanced, slightly discontented. Or we develop addictions to try and fill the hole inside. This hole is not empty, it is just that our society hasn't developed a useful way to teach our children (or our adults) how to access the spiritual side.

Some of us may become overly emotional and feel overwhelmed, as if we have no control. We think we are victims and so avoid what we are really feeling. 'Why is this happening to me?' 'It's not fair.' 'Everyone is against me.'

Alternatively, the soul might try and reach us through our rational conscious mind – 'I'm not happy in this job' might be the thought. Again we try and rationalise such thoughts away. 'I need the money.' 'I should be happy, it's a very good job.' 'I'm good at the job and I don't know what else I could do.'

Or we start trying to bargain with ourselves. 'I only have to do this job for another five years, then the children will have finished school and...' Or 'I only have to work for another seven years and I'll be eligible for superannuation/long service/retirement.'

Our soul might give us a message through our physical body leading to physical symptoms. Usually these are small things at first, like a dose of the flu so we must lie around and have a break from our busy lives, or a troublesome sore knee, or maybe a pain in the back or neck. Then something bigger that demands we pay more attention – chest pain, severe headaches or a broken leg. We tell ourselves that such physical problems arise from things outside of ourselves and we go to experts to have them fixed.

Our inner self might send us messages that all is not right in our world through our right brain and our intuition, through our dreams, our gut feelings, and through other signs.

Our souls might sometimes send us messages through other people and things. Have you heard the same song five times today? What might the lyrics have to say to you? Does that bumper sticker have a particular message for you? Is that phone call from your friend telling you anything?

The inner self can try to get us to pay attention through these five aspects of ourselves: feelings, thoughts, physical symptoms, intuition, and our interconnections,[6] but we have got so good at shutting ourselves off from our souls that it may take a truck to make us pay attention.

Some of us get hit by trucks, often metaphorically but sometimes literally.

The person who is diagnosed with cancer and suddenly realises that the life they have been living is not the life they were meant to be living. The person whose heart attack makes them realise that the important things in their life are not money and power but their family and friends. The person who gets chronic fatigue and is forced to re-evaluate their whole life.

Trucks are for those of us who live so out of touch with our spiritual self that the only way to get us to pay attention is to ram a truck right into us. For me, there were two big trucks. The first was when my marriage collapsed, the second when Angela died. Soon after Angela died, I began to understand why our soul sometimes needs to send us messages in a truck. It is because many of us just aren't paying attention to our inner selves. We are only paying attention to our left brain. So in 2004, I finally began to pay attention to my life's process. The process happens when our inner self tries to enter our conscious awareness.

I quit my main job and followed where my soul was pulling me. Around the same time, in that wonderful synchronistic way that the world works, my parents gave me a large sum of money. This meant I could concentrate on writing this book, which I had unsuccessfully been trying to start for a couple of years. Everything seemed to fall into place.

I began this book with no idea of what to write, just a relentless urge to write. I roughly mapped out a plan but as I began to write the plan disappeared. The whole book was written mostly from a

---

6   This aspect will be discussed further later in this chapter.

place deep inside of me that is usually not consciously available. As I wrote I began to understand how all the experiences I had had, and that I was still having, were helping me write.

I would be stuck on a concept or a chapter and then something would happen in my life that would suddenly make sense and enable me to continue. It was as if I was learning to listen to my own soul and in the process write a book about it. For a long time I had great plans for this book until I realised that I had to write it for myself most of all.

Our inner self speaks to us in many ways. Even when we aren't conscious of its presence, it is speaking to us. As we become more conscious of its presence we can begin to pay attention to how it talks. There are messages from our inner self in our feelings, our intuition, in signs and dreams, from our thoughts and our physical symptoms and via the connections between us all. The trouble is we don't understand the language most of the time because it doesn't make logical sense to us.

Holistic health model

This model is a representation of a holistic reality, yet I have to explain it in physical terms because this is how we communicate. There are many layers to this model and it is not truth, it just represents my version of how things might work, a metaphor to understand ourselves better. This understanding helps us move towards wholeness, but any model will change as we transform. Models of how the world works have a limited shelf life because the world is forever changing.

There are layers of the model but to begin, we start with the basics.

At the most basic level we are made up of two parts – our physical self (mind-body) and our spiritual self. In holistic terms imagine that we are like the yin and yang symbol – part of mind-body is spirit and part of spirit is mind-body. We can look at the physical and the spiritual as separate but really, they can't be separated – holistically they are combined, but as we live in what appears to be a physical world they appear to be two parts.

Our ego filters information coming into our consciousness. The information comes from the external world via our senses (vision, hearing, taste, smell, and touch) but it also comes from our inner world (soul and spirit). The ego processes all the incoming information and tries to decide what is truth or reality (or more accurately what it believes to be truth or reality). We live our lives based upon our ego's interpretations and decisions.

In Western society, ego (our conscious awareness) relies more on the external messages than the internal. But our soul is always trying to get our attention. It is always sending our conscious mind messages from our subconscious and unconscious self. It seems that when we came to earth as babies, all the knowledge and wisdom of our spirit self was hidden from us, from our conscious mind (the mind we think with, the mind that chatters away and makes our decisions). This wisdom of our inner self is not immediately accessible to our conscious thinking brain, but it is accessible and the more we understand how it works the more we can understand ourselves.

Our inner self sends messages through our elemental processes – air, fire, water, and earth.

This is what might be called the basic content of the model – the parts, except that there is one more part – ether. Ether is by its very nature ethereal, it is the element that is unworldly, spiritual, immaterial, intangible. This element is very difficult to fully describe but it symbolises the connections between our parts and the connections between us and everything else. It is the energy that is at the basis of all life but it is not simply energy, it is connections. I will explain this more fully in Part two.

The element of ether is the element of possibilities, the realm where anything can happen, even miracles. When we become aware of this element in our lives we begin to see possibilities where before we saw nothing. We begin to take notice of the world around us and how we fit into it. We begin to notice that when the weather is grey we often feel grey, that when the moon is full we feel more emotional, that the song that keeps playing on the radio has some sort of message for us. We notice that our interactions with other people and things are influenced by our energy, and vice-versa. We notice that we can feel happy by being with others who are happy or that we can feel sad just because someone we love is sad.

There is no logic to it. The connection between us all exists because we are all connected.

Some would call this etheric element God or The Divine or All That Is. Some would call it the Holy Spirit or the Web of Life or the quantum hologram. Some would call it Mother Nature or Gaia. This element that I have called ether is so much a part of everything that we cannot distil it out to discover its nature. We cannot reduce living things to all their parts and call one of these parts ether and expect to then understand what this means. Because ether more than anything is present most in the harmonic combination of the parts.

We have five parts or elements.

As well as the parts there is movement. As well as content, life has a process – it moves. There are no constants in life, it is always

Spirit

Air

Water

Earth

Fire

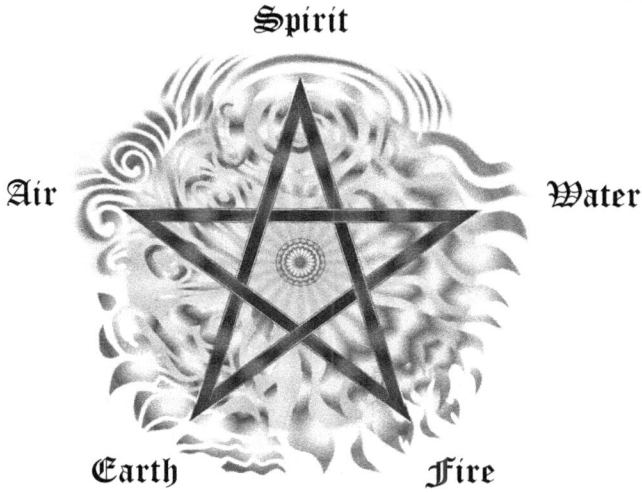

moving. This is embodied in the Taoist yin yang symbol. The fluid edge between the two indicates the constant movement of life. As yin expands, yang recedes. As yang expands, yin recedes. Life is the constant movement between the two.

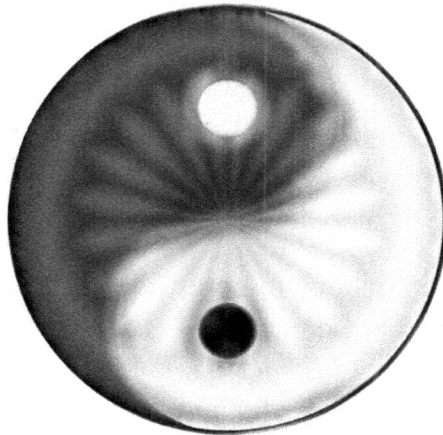

Our inner self uses the process of our life to try to catch our conscious attention. This inner spiritual self works in ways we don't understand to direct us to a greater awareness. Everything that happens to us is part of spirit's attempt to increase our individual consciousness and help us live whole lives.

The path we follow, the process our lives undergo, is orchestrated by our own spirit, which in holistic terms is an integral part of the whole universe and beyond. This means that we can stop agonising over where we are going in our lives and just live what is happening now. We can stop worrying about everyone else's path and leave them to live it, knowing their inner self is in control. (I find this hard to do; it is easier for us all to see how other people might grow than to see it in ourselves.) We can learn to trust the process. This is a major step in our transformation towards living a whole life.

Trust the process of life.

Trust that the life your Self is creating is perfectly designed to help you learn how to become more fully aware of your potential. And trust that it is so for every other person. This is the dance of life and it is individually created.

Our Self is guiding the process of our life, creating the life that we need in order for us to become conscious that who we really are is something beyond our physical self. Once we can grasp this and let soul guide us, we can begin to live the life we were meant to live.

It is a mistake to believe that this process has an endpoint. It is a mistake to think that being whole is a static thing that one day we reach. Wholeness is a tricky combination of integrating our parts and living our process. The parts are always changing and the process is ongoing. The dancing never stops.

THREE –
TRUE OR FALSE?

B eliefs are thoughts we hold in our minds that determine how we perceive the world and everyone in it.

Our beliefs are not truth or fact or reality, they are simply our current version of truth and reality.

Who we think we are is made up of a set of beliefs we hold.

How we think the world to be is made up of a set of beliefs we hold.

Our whole experience of life is based upon a set of beliefs.

For many years everyone believed the world to be flat. People believed this to be a fact – truth. Once it was discovered the world was round people had to give up their belief in flatness.

We laugh at this belief now but how many of our beliefs are similarly flawed? We really don't know. Many things we believe to be truth or reality turn out upon further investigation to not be truth.

None of what I write about is necessarily truth – it is just my beliefs about truth and reality. All of our beliefs are restricted by both a lack of knowledge and a lack of perception.

We don't know everything and we don't perceive everything. We are mostly restricted to perceiving what is in the three-dimensional world we live in.[7] The paradox is that we cannot perceive the dimensions we don't believe or know to exist, so we believe they can't exist.

When we believed that the world was flat, all the evidence we collected pointed to this as being true. Once we opened ourselves up to the possibility that the world was round, we discovered that it was. Here we are on the edge of another flat world, a firmly held belief in the science of logic and the physical. We limit ourselves to the three-dimensional reality when it is possible that the only limiting factor is our belief system.

Are our minds open to other possibilities and therefore open to other evidence, or are they shut?

Can we see that our beliefs about reality are just beliefs, or do we have to maintain them as truth?

Dualism

Dualism is the idea that there are two opposite forces in the world. The opposing forces might be good and evil but more commonly, we believe something to be right or wrong, true or false. So when we take a dualistic approach to a problem, we believe there is an answer that is right or wrong. This type of black and white thinking is the domain of the left brain; it is part of the linear process. Our left brain measures everything using a two-dimensional measure. Our judgements about right and wrong are made using our left brain.

Our left brain actually believes in absolutes. Things can be absolutely right or absolutely wrong because it measures things in only two dimensions. This is the only way it can think. This is a very

---

7　The physical world is made up of three dimensions of space (depth, width and height), and one dimension of time (now), although even this is just one world view. Einstein considered it a space-time continuum.

important thing to understand about ourselves. Our left brain, our logical thinking, can only think in lines. It uses that process. It cannot think in wholes, it can only think in parts of wholes. Even when it tries to put all the parts together, the left brain can never fully understand the whole. It can never see the woods, only the trees. This is not a fault within the left brain, it is simply how it processes information.

When we rely upon rational thinking to solve problems, we can never see the whole problem, only the bits. We can never reach a full understanding of any whole thing using only our left brain.

Because our society and most of us favour this type of left-brain thinking over the holistic process of the right brain, we like to divide everything in a dualistic way. It makes things seem simpler to us – and they are. Yet when we explain things dualistically, we never see the whole picture, only the parts.

When we take a dualistic view of the world, it affects our beliefs about ourselves and about the world we live in. There are always two ends of a line and so we make judgements based upon two extremes. This is how we come up with the idea (belief) that something is good or bad, right or wrong, true or false.

The left brain has a ruler that it measures everything with, or maybe a pair of scales is a more accurate metaphor. It measures out the evidence for one side and the evidence for the other. It decides which is right by the weight of the evidence. It only ever sees the two sides as opposing.

The right brain sees a sphere and measures everything by how balanced the sphere is. It is only interested in the balance, not in the reasons why. Even this isn't accurate because we live in a four-dimensional world (three of space and one of time) and there may be more dimensions we are unaware of. Let's imagine that the right

45

brain assesses everything by using a sphere and all it is interested in is keeping the sphere balanced. To the right brain, right and wrong have no meaning except in how they balance our sphere.

Now our whole person is closer to a sphere than to the left brain's scales. If we want to develop this further we might imagine that the whole person is like the earth. A perfect orb in the middle of a giant universe. All the earth needs to do in order to be itself is to keep in balance. The things that affect this balance are all the systems within it and all the systems around it.

So it is with humans. We are like small planets simply trying to stay in balance. Our balance is affected by what goes on inside us and outside of us.

Remember this is a three-dimensional representation of something that is more complex than this. At least it is an advance on a two-dimensional representation, which is what the left brain would have us believe is reality.

We have been taught and we continue to teach our children to shut the ego bridge to almost all traffic except that coming through the filter of our left brain. So our conscious awareness (which is who we believe we are) is full of left-brain thinking processes.

Luckily, our inner self and all our parts that we are not yet consciously aware of are struggling to get through our ego and over the bridge into our consciousness. This is our constant struggle. This is why our lives are so full of struggle because our real self, our whole self, is not being expressed physically.

The beliefs we hold in our mind, in our conscious awareness, are therefore largely a product of the left brain in Western society. They are not truth even though we think they are. We hold onto them because it feels safe, and it feels safe because if we believe that life is two-dimensional then we can control it.

This is a reassuring thought – that we can control life. This is what we would all like to believe and what we convince ourselves is truth. That we are in control and that the control we have operates in a linear fashion. When we encounter a problem, we believe that there is a right answer to it. We believe this because it makes us feel safe. We believe this because the left brain believes this, that because everything is two dimensional we can control it.

If everything is two dimensional then it might be possible for us to control it.

But life has more than two dimensions.

Rather than observing the world and understanding that we do live in a four-dimensional reality, we try to fit the world into two dimensions, we try to understand the world through our left brain's way of seeing. Our left brain cannot see beyond two dimensions. It simply can't. It isn't that the left brain is stupid or stubborn, it is just that it can't see beyond a line. Remember this is a model. It may not be strictly true that the left brain can't see beyond a line but it helps us understand the two ways of thinking – linear (the left brain) and non-linear (right brain).

As most of us process new information through the filter of our left brain, I am trying to write about it in terms that the left brain understands – dualistic terms. Remember, the left brain can't totally understand holism, it can only understand the parts. It can't see the wood for the trees. It can't see the whole for the parts. Let's at least make sure it can see all the parts.

In dualistic terms, my model begins with the two halves – light and dark, spiritual and physical, yang and yin. The spiritual can be divided into two parts – air and fire (both of which have yang tendencies), and the physical can be divided into two – earth and water (which have yin tendencies).

Of course, ether is part of the mix as well so each part is connected to each other part.

Holism as dualism model A

Ether

Physical self	**Spiritual self**
Earth	Fire
Water	Air

Ego is the other ingredient and it sits as the bridge between our inner self and our conscious awareness. In Western society, ego is most closely aligned with the physical self so we believe ourselves to be physical beings when we are both physical and spiritual.

Balance comes when our spiritual and physical sides are balanced and our ego sits between the two. We are consciously aware of both parts in balance. Remember however, that this is a two-dimensional representation of a much more complex system.

Holism as dualism model B

Ether
Ego (conscious awareness)

Physical self	**Spiritual self**
Earth	Fire
Water	Air

The qualities of each element are not fixed. While in the west we like to categorise everything into right and wrong, good and bad, etc., essentially we cannot do this. Everything is relative to everything else.

We begin with yang and yin and we might say that yang is our spiritual self and yin is our physical self. Or we might decide to call yin our spiritual self and yang our physical self. It actually depends on which way we are looking. Typically, yang is seen as light and therefore spiritual. We have a tendency to grow towards the light. Yin is the dark. Some cultures however might consider the dark to be the spiritual dimension and the light the physical dimension. It doesn't matter because when we get to the bottom of it, the physical and the spiritual are the same. However, let's leave that theory to part three.

Air by itself would be classified as yang.[8] If however we look at air relative to fire, it would be seen as yin. If we look at it relative to earth, it would again be yang. More about this in the next part. It is enough to remember that no part of the human system can ever be understood on its own. We only fully understand the parts when we see how they relate to other parts and other people.

Content and process

So far, I have concentrated on the parts of the human system in much the same way that mechanistic science reduces a system to its parts to attempt to understand it. However, this only gives us an understanding of the content of the system. The content of the human system is the parts.

---

8   However, holistic traditions would never try to look at something like air in isolation. It is always related and connected to everything else.

The other aspect of every system is the process. This is what keeps the system in motion. The left brain likes to divide the content and process into separate categories. It assumes that we can approach them separately (dualistically). But content and process are always connected.

Two main processes occur – the linear process and the non-linear process. The linear process is the one we are most familiar with – cause and effect. The non-linear process (or chaotic process) has no cause and effect line (thus, 'non-linear'). In chaos, there is process and outcome but the process doesn't follow a line, it goes anywhere. I will explain these processes further. For now, all I need you to conceptualise is that the whole self is made up of these various parts and that it is dancing along to the processes of life.

It is very difficult to draw a model that encompasses content and process because process has a dimension in time, a movement. We can describe these ideas in words and try to visualise them in models and pictures in our heads, but true understanding is about processing the knowledge into understanding.

We begin by trying to understand the pieces and the concepts – the tangible parts of ourselves that go to make up the more complex system.

We become aware of the dual nature of our self, our physical and spiritual aspects, and we begin to see ourselves as complex systems (within a larger system). We stop identifying the self as our thoughts or our body or only those parts of ourselves that we are conscious of. We learn to balance our spiritual needs and our physical needs. We learn about how balancing our parts and living the process of our lives brings us to a greater understanding of ourselves and of the greater system. We learn this wisdom not from books but by living the process of our lives in a conscious way. We pay attention to what happens to us.

As we grow in consciousness, we become aware of holism – that the physical and spiritual are essentially the same. We begin to transcend the individual self and know instead that we are one with everything else, yet at the same time separate. None of these stages is like levels that we suddenly achieve. It is more like a gradual process of unfolding and a letting go of dualism. As we do this, we move into wholeness, which is our natural state.

This book is concerned with all of these stages.

Parts one and two deal with the parts of the system – the content (and its parts) and the processes. They also attempt to help people understand that all of our beliefs are open to challenge. When we can challenge the basis of our lives (our belief system), we can begin to differentiate from our belief that our identity lies in our brain or our ego.

Part three of the book looks at the theory behind the holistic approach and tries to help the left brain better understand holism and the science behind it.

Part four looks at the stage when we become aware of our dual nature and shows how we might follow the process of our lives to learn more about who we are and how we fit into the greater system. This is the healing journey.

FOUR -
CONTENT AND PROCESS

Having looked at the basic content of the human system, we now turn to look at the processes that govern the system. Two basic processes drive the process of life.[9] The first is the linear process. This is the process that both the left brain and Western society love. The second is the non-linear or chaotic process.

Linear processes

A linear process is a process that takes the path of a line. It can be described and graphed in two dimensions. Typically, it might describe one aspect of growth, such as the height of a child over time. The growth as measured by height is graphed against time and the resulting line shows the child's growth. We call this a linear process – it may be a straight line or a curved line but essentially it is a line.

Linear processes are usually more complex but the basis of them is that the outcome can be predicted based on a set number of factors. If we know what the factors are, we can predict what the outcome will be. The process travels in a line.

We see this type of process occurring in pure left-brain thinking. We have a problem; we take into account all the factors and come up with an answer. A purely mathematical problem is solved by

9   Of course there are more processes, many as yet undiscovered, but for the purposes of this book I will keep it simple.

linear thinking. Much of Western scientific and economic belief is based upon the idea that linear processes rule the physical world. We believe that if we know enough we can predict outcomes.

Indeed, for most linear processes we can predict the outcomes if we know all the relevant variables that affect the process.

If we can work out all the variables that make it likely someone will have a heart attack, then we can alter the inputs and therefore change the outcome. Science decides that the predisposing factors are smoking, high cholesterol, high blood pressure, diabetes, family history, and being male.[10] So medicine decides that if we get everyone to stop smoking, lower their cholesterol and their blood pressure and get them fit, then the rate of heart attacks will decrease.

This is a typical linear scientific method based upon our knowledge of the linear process.

There are a number of problems with this.

The first is that we never know all the variables in the process; science is continually finding more of them.

The second is that some of the variables can't be changed, gender and age being two variables that we have little control over.

The third is that some of the variables that make us more likely to have a heart attack might make us less likely to have some other illness. Science and medicine are continually chasing their tails trying to work out the perfect lifestyle to avoid heart attacks, every type of cancer, stroke, traffic accident, suicide, and arthritis. We are

---

10   This is not the whole story – there are other factors, but science and medicine are always playing the odds. The odds are that if you are a sixty-year-old overweight male, you smoke and have high cholesterol and high blood pressure, and your father died of a heart attack in his fifties, your chance of having a heart attack is much greater than a for-ty–year-old female who is healthy and doesn't smoke and whose parents are both alive.

a very complex system and our health does not simply rely upon getting every variable under control.

The fourth problem with the linear scientific method in medicine is that the outcome that all medicine attempts to prevent is death. We also want to prevent ill health, but preventing death seems to be our highest priority. This is a fine aim, however we must understand that the linear process always ends in death no matter what. Death is always the outcome of life.

Science has made many advances in learning how to have some measure of control over linear processes.

If we know all the relevant variables that affect the strength of a bridge, we can build a bridge that will withstand the amount of traffic we have built it to carry.

If we know more about the basics for healthy living, we can live longer. The basics of clean drinking water, sufficient healthy food and good sanitation have saved more lives and increased life expectancy more than any medical treatments.

But there is something else going on; life is not just linear. We have been under the illusion that because time seems to travel in a straight line, our lives follow only this linear process.

Non-linear processes

The second type of process in life is the non-linear process or the chaotic process.

This is the realm of chaos theory. Non-linear processes are also called chaotic because they do not follow the same logical rules of linear processes – they are chaotic in nature.

I am not a physicist or a mathematician so my view of Chaos theory is a little limited, but it will do for now. For a more thorough explanation, I recommend you read Chaos by James Gleick.[11]

Chaos is the study of non-linear processes. Chaos is based upon the discovery that many complex systems do not operate under a linear process. That is, no matter whether or not you know all the factors in the system, you cannot predict the outcome because the process is non-linear or 'chaotic'.

In a non-linear or chaotic system, the process does not follow a line. Rather, the process can go anywhere, and it often does. It isn't that a chaotic process doesn't reach an outcome, but the outcome cannot be predicted in the same way the outcome of a linear process can be predicted.

Similarly, if the outcome cannot be predicted, altering the variables that go into the system cannot predictably alter the outcome. We might alter the variables but we have no idea what this will do to the outcome of the process. In a linear system when we alter the variables, we have a fairly good idea what effect this will have on the outcome. Not so in a chaotic system.

Let me illustrate how a chaotic process might occur. Remember this is an illustration or metaphor for a chaotic process.

I believe that my house should be neat and orderly, but the state of my house reflects the fact that it is not just a house but a home, a system with many variables that go in to make up the system. It operates under the natural laws of chaos.

So I clean the house and then the people who live in the house re-enter the system. The dog sheds white hair on the couch. Emma drops her school bag right where everyone walks and kicks her

11   Details in Bibliography.

shoes off. Sarah drops her school bag next to Emma's and kicks her shoes off. I kick my shoes off. Kate puts her bag in her room and places her shoes in the place she thinks they should go. She yells at us for being messy. Emma and Sarah raid the kitchen and take the food into the lounge room, leaving various containers on the bench. Kate does the same but moves to the table where she spreads out her homework.

Gradually the effects of chaos make themselves known.

The house begins to resemble a disaster area and we can't find the table. We also can't find the car keys or Emma's left shoe. This is the height of the process of chaos. Everything is in disarray and all seems hopeless but somehow, the various aspects of the system that is our home come to our awareness.

For a time we each blame the other parts of the system. I kick the dog out of the house, Kate yells at Emma for leaving her bag right where she tripped over it. Emma is upset because she still can't find her shoe. Sarah retires to her room because it is all too much.

Then the beauty of the chaos system reveals itself. Just when we thought the whole house would disappear under the chaos, each part of the system begins to realise that it is part of a system and that therefore we are the only people who can make a difference. Each of us, except perhaps the dog, begins to play a part in recreating order.

As this happens, the order that we create is different in some way from the order that went before. Kate decides to move the shoe spot to a place where all of us will actually put our shoes. Emma decides that Kate is right and that she needs to put her bag away in her room. I clean up my mess, which leads Sarah to clean up hers. Kate sees that Emma is making an effort so Kate offers to help her with her room. The house becomes cleaner and more orderly and we all learn something about how this system that is our home works better. We create a better home. We create it by restoring it to its wholeness not simply by cleaning it. The new wholeness (sense of order) is slightly better than the old one.

This is the beauty of the process of chaos; it is always pushing the system towards wholeness. Wholeness is that state where all the parts of the system are working together for the good of the system (which is also the good of the parts.) The system is in harmony.

Of course, this same process of chaos happens every week in our house and ever so gradually the system begins to work better. We become a whole system. However, the process of chaos and the expression of wholeness are always inhibited by those parts of the system that believe they know the right answer. Typically, this is me because I am the mother, or Kate because she is the first-born daughter and a Virgo. Alternatively, one or other of us will take over the running of the system. We will try to run it along linear lines. We will make rules about what goes where and who does what and how this house will run. We try to turn a naturally chaotic system into a linear system and it can't be done without forgoing wholeness. When any system forgoes wholeness, the process of chaos ensues. This natural process is designed to return the system to wholeness.

More recently, our home has erupted into more chaos because some parts of the system have decided they are not part of the system. Instead, they are teenagers trying to undergo the process of individuation and separation. In many ways, they are trying to escape the system they have been born into. They are trying to discover where they fit into the bigger system. I find myself attempting to reinstitute rules and regulations in order to regain control and go back to the good old days when my children were happier to be told what to do. But we cannot return to the good old days, we can only grow and learn.

In a physically orientated culture, we are obsessed with outcomes and control. We want to know exactly where we are going and how we are going to get there. We think if we can control everything around us, we can control all the outcomes. This type of thinking is linear and arises in our left brain. We believe that the cause of something directly affects the result (or that the result is directly attributable to the cause). When the process of our life challenges this belief system, we get confused.

We base our life on the incorrect assumption or belief that life only follows this linear process. This is basic science; this is the basis of rational, scientific thought. We believe that we can work out all our problems through a linear process. If we do x and y we will get z. If I am good and work hard, I will be happy. If I do what God wants, I will go to heaven. If I control my thoughts, I can affect the outcome. If my daughters follow the rules for a clean house then we will have a happy home.

Cause and effect. If you drink and drive, you will have an accident. If you smoke, you will get lung cancer. If you eat too much, you will be overweight.

Our whole lives are based upon this belief in the linear process, in cause and effect. We are always looking for causes in the hope we can have an effect on an outcome.

Here is another point where holism (and holistic medicine) diverges from rational scientific thought and Western medicine.

In life there is often no cause and effect. Life is not really linear. This is an illusion.

There is balance and imbalance, harmony or disharmony. Chaos ensues when a system loses its harmony, and chaos is the process by which harmony is restored. Harmony is wholeness. Wholeness is not some fixed point or sense of order. Wholeness is when all the parts of the system are in harmony with each other part. Part of every living system is movement, so that balance is not a fixed point (as on a scale that measures weight) but an ever-changing dance. Chaos seems to me to be nature's way of restoring the balance of yin and yang. It does not have a cause per se but it happens when the balance of yin and yang goes too far one way. We call it chaos because that's what it feels like, but really, yin or yang is dominant and life must swing the other way. Yang dominates and we have too much activity and growth, which leads to death in the cycle, and then yin flows back and things can be reborn and the cycle continues.

Holistic culture appreciates that life mostly follows a chaotic process, which means appreciating that we cannot control the outcome in linear ways. We learn about the process itself. There are ways to have control over this process but we are only now discovering them, for we are learning how to undergo the process. By undergoing the process, we allow ourselves to return to our wholeness and to participate in the cycles of life.

We are effectively, at this stage in our evolution, coming to grips with chaotic processes and how we might live them better. We once believed the earth was flat and then we discovered it was round. We once believed that life was a straight-line process and now we discover it has more dimensions than that. Interestingly, it seems that we have come full circle from the traditional native cultures, who viewed the world holistically. What have we learnt in the process? Have we come full circle? Or is it more like an evolutionary spiral, where the lessons of living the process of life are being taken from an isolated tribal context to a whole of earth context?

Linear thinking

I hope I have shown how most of our belief systems are based upon linear processing and left-brain thinking. These belief systems are inherently limited because they limit us to linear dimensions. To live more easily in a world ruled by chaos we need to learn how chaos works. Yet most of us keep trying to control chaos with our linear thinking.

In Western society, there are three main variants of our linear beliefs. Most of us use a combination of all three.

The first is the religious belief system. Here the linear thinking goes something like:

'If I do God's will and follow all his rules (inputs) I will go to heaven' (outcome).

'If I am a good person I will live a good life.'

'If I am a spiritual person I will be rewarded.'

The second is the scientific or logic belief system. Here the linear thinking goes something like:

'If I work out logically what I want to do and where I want to go in my life and do the 53 things required to get there then I will achieve my goal.'

'I want to get married and have children (goal) so if I work out exactly how to do that (action) it will happen for me (outcome).'

'If I eat healthily, stop smoking, exercise regularly, have two yearly pap smears, meditate, and have loving relationships I will live longer.'

The third is the magical belief system. This is the current new age favourite. This goes along the lines of:

'If I control my thoughts and visualise exactly what I want in my life I can manifest it.'

'If I visualise and affirm that I want a million dollars and I believe this and take some action to also affirm it then I can get it.'

We are entrenched in our left-brain ways of thinking and processing. All of these are limiting beliefs simply because they limit us to try to control linear processes when most of life also follows chaotic processes. These belief systems keep us entrenched in our belief that there is always a cause and therefore always an effect, and that somehow we can (either by God, intellect or through the power of the mind) control the effect or somehow influence the cause.

For each of us, the primary difference between linear and chaotic processes is that in a chaotic process we cannot control or predict the outcome. We must always enter into the process to see where it takes us.

Riddle

How do you make God Laugh?

Tell him your plans.

We persist in thinking that we can plan our life and that it will go according to our plans – this is typical of the left brain and the way it thinks. The left brain is cleverly designed to help us with linear problems; it is not so good with non-linear problems. Luckily, we have our right brain to help us sort through our non-linear problems, but most of us in Western society have forgotten how useful it is.

Imagine that you are married and that you fall in love with another married person. Let's imagine that you are Barry and you have fallen in love with Linda who is married to Roger. You have been married to your wife Renee for seven years and you have two children. Renee also has a child from a previous marriage who lives with her ex-husband. Linda has three children and works as a nurse in the local hospital.

You (Barry) work in real estate and meet Linda and Roger at a party with mutual friends. The four of you get along well and you discover that you both have a child who has just started at the same school. You also discover that you and Linda grew up in the same town and went to the same school.

As you get to know each other over a number of months you realise that you are developing strong feelings for Linda but you pretend to yourself that you don't have these feelings or that they are symptoms of the seven-year itch. Gradually you come to realise that Linda has similar feelings.

You enter a state of confusion where you have no idea what to do. Your mind tries to work out what you *should* do, what is the *right* thing to do. The occasion arises where the two of you are together alone and despite all your best intentions, you end up kissing Linda and she returns the kiss. 'What are we going to do?' you ask each other. 'This is crazy,' you say, 'this doesn't make any sense.'

You both go home feeling guilty but with a secret fire inside. Linda understands you in a way that Renee no longer does. You have a connection that you can't just ignore.

You may go in many directions at this point – you may decide to have an affair and spend secret time with Linda while maintaining the illusion that your marriage is okay. You may tell Renee about your feelings for Linda or decide to tell Linda you can't see her any more, or many other variations.

Let's say you tell your wife Renee. She throws a plate at you and storms out, taking the kids with her. She rings Roger and tells him what is happening. Linda rings you in tears telling you that Roger is upset and angry. Everything escalates.

This is part of the chaotic process.

This is the process of life and it happens all the time.

When it happens we usually try to look at it logically and say, 'Well Barry shouldn't have fallen in love with Linda', as if we can control love.

Or we might look at it from a religious point of view and say, 'Barry shouldn't have acted on his impulses' or 'Barry shouldn't have even thought about coveting his neighbour's wife.'

Or we could look at it from a magical belief system, which would say that if Barry can visualise the outcome he wants then he can have that outcome.

None of these approaches solves the problem because they all take a linear approach to a chaotic process.

Unfortunately, science isn't much help here either because science hasn't learnt how to control chaotic processes. In fact, one of the things about chaotic processes is that they exhibit a lack of control (as we understand control in linear terms).

So what happens to Barry and Linda and Renee and Roger? Well, they all enter this chaotic process and if they are willing to undergo personal change and take a deeper meaning from the process then they come out the other end more whole people. If they are not willing to undergo the process, it's still going to happen. If they choose to pursue their limited beliefs about what should happen and what other people involved should do, they will come out the other end hurt, angry and bitter.

Fortunately, most of these wonderful chaotic processes serve to make us more aware of our limiting beliefs and more able to let them go. In all these chaotic processes, something has to give, hopefully, our limited beliefs.

How do we have any measure of control over the process of chaos? We give up the idea that we can control it with logic, God or magic (linear thinking). We allow our intuitive thinking to guide us. Intuitive thinking after all is based upon non-linear processes. This type of thinking is most likely to help.

Intuitive thinking happens when we stop trying to control things. The outcome is not pre-determined, the outcome is not predictable, and the outcome cannot be controlled.

Let me repeat that – the outcome cannot be controlled.

When we are in chaos, we cannot control the outcome, at least not in the logical linear way we have learnt. In non-linear processes, there is no such thing as cause and effect. There is no cause and there is no effect.

It is of course possible that in using our intuitive thinking, we can influence the outcome but this is not a cause and effect influence. We cannot decide on the outcome and work towards it. A linear process would work this way. We can allow our intuitive mind to help us reach the outcome more quickly. The outcome we probably want is for the process of chaos to be over. We always want to reach an outcome.

Barry wants to stop being confused and uncomfortable. Typically, Barry tries to work out what outcome he wants and then tries to work out how he will get there.

He might decide he wants to stay with Renee and that he won't see Linda any more. Renee, however, is not so sure about this. She isn't sure whether she wants to stay with someone who has betrayed her trust, she needs time to sort things out for herself. Barry is convinced that what he wants is his old life back so he tries everything he knows to get it back, but nothing works. Renee decides to make the split permanent.

Then Barry might change his desired outcome and decide he wants to get together with Linda, but by now she and Roger have rediscovered their love for each other and gone off on a second honeymoon.

Barry clearly has no control here.

If he were able to let go of his need for control (which is very difficult for all of us) and tap into his intuition, then he may find some answers that he never even knew had questions.

He may find that his relationship with Renee was lacking something. He may find that he hasn't been satisfied with his work life. He may find that he hasn't had a fulfilling relationship with his children and that now they are not around he has realised the importance of them in his life. He may also realise that this degree of chaos might have been avoidable if he had only listened to himself better in the first place.

The process of chaos brings to our conscious awareness many things that we have been unconscious of. Primarily, it brings to our awareness (if we let it) how we have forgotten some parts of ourselves, forgotten who we really are and what is really important in our lives, how we have become fragmented. Chaos is the process by which life attempts to heal us, and by undergoing it, we learn how to become whole.

We see this process all around us in nature. Chaos is the destruction of a storm or an earthquake or a hurricane. The outcome of such destruction is always a bringing together of parts, a reunification. Not just of the physical environment (although this is part of it) but of the world as a whole. It is the process of healing, in the sense that chaos attempts to return the system to wholeness and order. But wholeness and order are always changing; the system does not go back to its previous wholeness and order, it goes forward to a new order, a new way of expressing its wholeness. Barry, Renee, Linda, Roger, and their families will not go back to their previous lives. They will go forward to something different. Our lives are always changing in response to the chaotic process. When we go with the process rather than fight against what we perceive is the unfairness of it, we have a better chance of finding out who we really are and how we fit into the world around us.

Part two looks in more detail at the parts of the human system and how they work.

THE ELEMENTS AND THE PROCESSES

Medicine is not only a science; it is also an art. It does not consist of compounding pills and plasters; it deals with the very processes of life, which must be understood before they may be guided.

Paracelsus

ONE - AIR

Our brain is divided into two hemispheres, the right and the left. In Part one, I wrote briefly about the difference between the two sides. The main difference is how they process information.

The left side is responsible for linear, logical, analytical thinking and is often called the 'intellectual' side.

The left brain thinks in lines. One thought follows another. The thoughts in our head might go something like this:

'I want something to eat. What do I feel like? Maybe some cake. No, that wouldn't be healthy, I shouldn't have cake. Well, I feel like it anyway. Oh, but Jake ate the last piece before. I'll have to go buy some. Maybe I should make it, that's what a good mum would do. No, that will take too much time. I want it now. Where are my car keys? And where is Jake, I'd better tell him I'm going.'

All of this happens very quickly. Most of us have a constant monologue or dialogue going on in our heads all the time. This is our left brain. This is what is often called the monkey mind because it chatters away like a monkey. It is a constant background noise. The right brain isn't still, it often chimes in with a picture or a symbol or an idea but it mostly doesn't think in words and sentences so we don't notice it so much.

The two sides are intimately connected, so intimately that we don't notice them as two different types of thinking. One reason to begin to take notice is that for many of us our left brain is so noisy that we forget to pay attention to our right. Our right brain thinks in a completely different way. It solves problems by looking at the whole problem, taking in all the information and arriving at an answer. This is our intuitive thinking. The right brain does not often think in word thoughts so we often assume it isn't doing any thinking.

Our right brain seems to find its answers without following a logical path, so we begin to doubt the answers it comes up with. This intuitive thinking is part of our intuitive sense, which doesn't lie solely in the brain.

Neither the left-brain process of rational thinking nor the right brain's intuitive thinking process is right or wrong. They are just different ways of reaching answers.

It is important to understand this difference between linear and non-linear thinking processes because it is where we often repeat our mistakes and get stuck in the same patterns of behaviour.

Many problems can be solved with linear thinking, but they have to be linear problems. Most of our problems, and certainly those we usually get stuck in, are non-linear. No-one can work them out with their left brain. Many people think they are stupid because they can't work out their problems. They go to a doctor or counsellor because they think such people are smarter.

The problem isn't smartness or lack of it; it is due to our reliance on a part of the brain that simply cannot solve these problems. The left brain cannot under any circumstances solve a non-linear problem. It is like trying to use a calculator for word processing, or a screwdriver to knock in a nail. It's just the wrong tool.

Our life is always trying to teach us this. When we find our brain going round and round in circles and not getting anywhere, we can be pretty sure our left brain is trying to sort out a non-linear problem.

It goes in circles but it never gets anywhere because the problem is not solvable through linear thought. The left brain can play a part in helping us through such problems but it cannot reach a solution by itself; it needs the help of the right brain.

Once we have learnt this lesson then we can turn to the part of our brain specifically designed for these non-linear problems, the right brain.

This is where we really enter the culture of the holistic because it is here that we change our belief system. We begin to believe that this process of right-brain thinking is the way to solve our non-linear problems. When I say solve I don't mean in a left-brain way, I mean in a holistic way.

The right brain helps us get to a different place. It helps us understand in an intuitive sense what is going on, what we have to learn, how we have to proceed. The problem is not linear or logical, therefore the process of solving it is not linear or logical, therefore the answer is not linear or logical. Intuitive answers do not always help us reach a predetermined outcome. Instead, they teach us more about ourselves, about reality, about how to be whole and how to live the cycles of life.

The answers from our right brain will not come to us by sitting down and thinking about the problem. Thinking, as we have come to know it, is how we define left-brain processing. Right-brain answers will usually come to us out of the blue, sometimes in a dream or as a sign or symbol. The beauty of right-brain thinking is that it doesn't make our head hurt like left-brain thinking can. We can just say, 'Okay right brain, here's the problem, take your time and give me the answer when you're ready. I'll be off having fun.' We can then go and do other things, leaving our right brain to sort things out and sure enough, eventually (or sometimes instantly), it will come back with the answer or the steps to take to find an answer.

Our lives would be easier if we would just leave a lot of our problems with our right brain and know that it can answer them for us.

The answers to all our problems are right there inside us. Most of us just look in the wrong place. We also expect them to come in a certain form when in a holistic world the answers are not often black and white, right or wrong. The answers are sometimes mysterious and require us to live with our problems until we reach clarity and understanding about why we ended up stuck again.

The process by which our intuition solves problems is non-linear (I know I am getting repetitive here). This means it doesn't make logical sense; you can't follow a line of thought from the problem to the solution. It is as if the right brain gathers all the available information (some of which is not available to our conscious thinking brain), puts it in a container, shakes it all up and then extracts the answer. The answer appears to have just popped into our heads but it popped in there because the right brain's intuitive non-linear processes made it available. This is how a chaotic process works. It begins and then there is what seems to be an utterly chaotic process and then an endpoint is reached. We cannot see or understand how the chaotic process resulted in an outcome.

We are not used to trusting the right brain's process of problem solving, partly because we can't make logical sense of it but also because we often don't like the answers we get. We can't make logical sense of intuitive processes because this is the essence of non-linear thinking – it's not logical.

I am being a bit extreme here to make a point and because so many patients I see are really stuck trying to 'work' out their problems. They forget that sometimes when we stop trying so hard to sort things out, the right side of the brain can come up with the answer.

Ultimately, we need to use both sides of our brain. The left side tries to take a problem apart and solve the parts, and the right side looks at the problem as a whole and tries to come up with a way forward. The left side needs the right side to see how the parts fit into the whole picture and the right side needs the left to see how the whole picture can be broken down into parts that are more manageable.

Too much logic

A 35-year-old man called Angus came to see me because his wife had left him for another man. He was angry and depressed. He couldn't sleep, eat or work. He felt that his life had collapsed around him. He couldn't speak to his wife because his anger was overwhelming. He couldn't bear the pain that she had inflicted on him but he could see no way out. He loved her and hated her at the same time. He wished she would come back to him or that he could move on with his life and not care about her.

Angus couldn't sleep because his mind was whirring away trying to find an answer. However, this is not a linear problem; there is no logic here, no rational explanation for what is happening. When we try to simplify such a situation to make it fit into our linear thinking, we end up more confused than ever.

The left brain can only solve left-brain problems, linear problems. Many of our problems are not linear. We become so confused and tie ourselves in mental knots because we persist in trying to use our left brain to help us.

Angus's problem is chaotic or non-linear in nature. There may be parts of it that his left brain can help sort out, but what he really needs in order to solve his problem is an understanding that the process he is going through is what he needs to go through to find his answers. He needs to stop thinking so much. This is a major shift in belief systems.

To move from the physical world view to the holistic world view requires this shift. We stop relying on our left brain to solve all our problems. We start to use our right brain more. We start to appreciate the messages from our body. We start to recognise that our feelings are important. But most of all we begin to appreciate that what is happening to us right now is what we need to learn about. What we are always learning about is who we really are and how we fit into the system.

Could Angus move from the frame of mind of 'My wife has left me, what am I going to do now, how can I get my old life back,' to a position of 'Okay let's see where this process is taking me'? This would be a major shift in the way that he thinks and acts.

The first hint of the shift is when a person recognises that the way they think is not helping. If Angus could recognise that his problem is not linear and therefore not soluble by his usual logical linear problem-solving processes, then he would start the shift.

For many of us, this major epiphany only occurs when we are so stuck in the middle of a problem that we can't find our way out. We are not in control the way we thought we were. Our intellect is not helping us in the way we are used to. We may feel like we are losing our mind and in a sense this is exactly what we need to do. Not to lose our mind literally but metaphorically. We need to lose the idea that our left brain can help us here. We need to lose that part of our controlling mind for a while in order to find our answers, or realise that sometimes the answers are not what we thought.

The occasions when we feel we are going crazy or that our brain won't stop thinking are yet another way the soul brings our hidden parts to our consciousness. When we get to this stage, we are able to say, 'I can't figure this out. My logical brain won't sort it out for me. I'm stuck. I don't know what to do.'

We then start to look for alternatives. Usually we go to doctors, counsellors or others to help us sort things out. We go to an expert to fix us because we believe that they are cleverer than us. The doctor will surely put their intellect (their superior left brain) to work to try to solve the problem. Many counsellors help the client to 'problem solve', or they use cognitive behaviour therapy. All of these still rely on left-brain processes. Our inner selves push us to stop relying solely on our left brain (or anyone else's left brain) to solve the problem. The left brain cannot sort the problem out on its own. Situations like these try to teach us to pay better attention to our other parts.

We have forgotten how to take advantage of the right side of our brain, which is useful at helping us sort out these types of problems.

Too little logic

While many of us rely too much on our linear thinking most of the time, we sometimes don't rely on it enough. Sometimes we forget how to use our linear thinking in useful ways and we keep trying to use it when it isn't working.

Our linear thinking works very well in situations where the process is linear and therefore logical, or where it can look at smaller parts of the process and work out a possible plan. Once the right brain has come up with a possible solution, the left brain is very good at planning out the steps required to get to that solution. It is also good at helping us work out why we are stuck at times.

Sometimes we are in a pattern of behaviour that always results in the same outcome. I nag my child to clean her room; she still does not clean her room. She feels grumpy with me for nagging; I feel grumpy at her for not cleaning her room and I blame her for making me nag. In this apparently linear process, my nagging does not have the required outcome of getting my child to clean her room.

If we look at it logically and linearly, my behaviour does not get the desired outcome and instead gets some undesired outcomes – everyone gets grumpier. Logically, I should therefore change the inputs. Remembering that I cannot control my child (because she is not a linear being but a chaotic system), I can only control my own behaviour (and often this I have difficulty with).

A linear process works in a straight-line way – the inputs lead to the outcome. This does not mean we can control the outcome by controlling the inputs, but it does mean the only way we can change an outcome is by changing the inputs.

My options in controlling the outcome of getting my child to clean her room are many – I just need to change my own inputs.

When something doesn't work, do something different. This is essential in a linear process (and often useful in a chaotic process).

I might try paying my child to clean her room, or cleaning it myself, or paying someone else to clean it. I need to be absolutely clear about my desired outcome. Is it for the room to be clean?

Or for the child to clean the room? Or for the child to become responsible?

When I have difficulty solving any problem, I might ask myself three questions:

1. What is my desired outcome?

2. Have I any measure of control over this outcome? (i.e. is this a linear process or a chaotic process?)

3. What can I change about my behaviour (my inputs)?

We only have a small measure of control in any event. We only have control over our own behaviour (even if most of us deny we can control this!). Changing our behaviour will change the outcome but not necessarily to the outcome we desire.

However, this is how we learn. We realise that what we are doing (how we are behaving) isn't working and we change it. We learn whether the change is useful or not. We learn that we can only change our own behaviour, not anyone else's. We learn that the outcome we desire is not always the outcome that we will get or the outcome that is in our best interests. But we change anyway because it is all we can do.

I decide that my desired outcome is that I would like my child's room not to be messy. Instead of nagging her, I just clean her room and I have my desired outcome.

I then learn that what I really wanted was for her to take responsibility for cleaning her room. Instead of nagging her, I give her the responsibility of cleaning her own room. She is responsible for her room, and if she chooses to have it messy, that is her responsibility.

I then learn that I can't necessarily have both outcomes – the room is her responsibility and the room is not messy.

This is how linear thinking can help us clarify some of our problems. We can use our logic to think our way through the problem, we can modify our behaviour, we can learn from the changes. This is an oversimplification but it helps us to understand how we often get stuck in the same old patterns without logically understanding why we are stuck.

We get stuck because we behave in exactly the same way and end up in exactly the same place.

We get stuck because we forget to change our behaviour in order to try to change the outcome.

We get stuck when we insist on a particular outcome and are unable to learn from the outcome we end up with.

We get stuck when we think we can have various outcomes that actually conflict with one another.

Six ways to help your mind

1. Don't expect the left brain to solve all your problems

As you learn that the left brain can only solve linear problems, you can let go of your expectation that it will fix everything for you. It simply can't. So when your problem feels chaotic and overwhelming and impossible to solve, you can be fairly sure that the problem is not linear and you can let your left brain have a rest.

You might need to tell yourself (or your left brain) that this is okay. It is okay that the left brain can't fix the problem. We don't get cross with a spanner if it can't act as a screwdriver. Yet we often get cross with our left brain when it can't fix things.

You need to say something like this to yourself (and you usually need to keep repeating it). 'This problem is not linear so I cannot solve it by thinking about it. My left brain, my logical thinking, simply cannot solve this problem. It is not that I am stupid or dumb it is just that I am trying to use my logic to solve a problem that is not logical. This is a waste of time and I will drive myself crazy if I keep doing it. When my thinking goes in circles it means that it is stuck and I just need to stop thinking so much.'

This is the motto for the holistic world view – stop thinking so much. As we let go of the need to think our way out of a problem logically, our right brain has a chance to kick in. I will talk more about this in Chapter four – Fire – which deals with our intuitive abilities, related to our right brain.

2. Give it a rest

To give your left brain a rest you may need to let it know that it is okay to take a rest. The temptation is to keep turning to your rational thinking. If only you think hard enough, you will find an answer. In fact, for non-linear problems the harder you think the more confused you become; you need to stop your left-brain thinking. You need to turn off your left brain or if you can't do that, you need to pay it less attention. Thoughts are just thoughts; you don't have to believe them or act on them. You can begin to let the thoughts go without giving them any power.

Some people rest their left brain through meditation or exercise or sleep. Some people try alcohol and drugs to sedate themselves. This is rarely necessary once you realise that the left brain is going crazy trying to do something it can't do. It pays to be aware that our drug use is often an attempt to stop our brains from thinking so much.

The right brain classically comes up with answers when our left brain is resting. So we might wake up with the answer, or find it in a dream or a daydream. It may just pop into our head when we are exercising or meditating. More about this in Chapter four.

3. Disengage your left brain

Until you learn how to rest the left brain, you might need to learn how to disengage it from ruminating on the problem. You disengage the left brain by engaging it on something else, thereby distracting it. Methods of distraction are many and varied but they usually work best if the left brain is given a job to do. Engage it in a serious linear problem and it will generally relax. The left brain does not like trying to sort out non-linear problems because it can't solve them; it goes in circles and drives itself crazy. Give it a linear problem to solve. The problem might be related to the non-linear problem (see 4 below) or it might be unrelated.

Writing all your thoughts down is sometimes a useful way of disengaging your thinking – not trying to solve problems, just recording the thoughts. This is why keeping a journal is so helpful. You can get your thoughts and feelings down on paper without having to judge them.

Alternatively, you can try observing your thoughts. Let them swirl around the left side of your brain without attaching yourself to them. Pretend your inner self is just observing the thoughts as they swirl around.

You don't have to stop your left brain from thinking. Rather, you learn how not to attach yourself to the thoughts. The thoughts are not the real us, they are just our left brain processing information.

While meditation is a good way of disengaging the left brain, often when we are in the throes of thinking too much, meditation is too hard. Instead, engage the left brain in something it likes doing. Word and number puzzles or games are ideal. They engage the left brain in useful work and as the left brain has trouble doing more than one thing at a time, this activity usually decreases the vortex of useless thinking that we get trapped in.

4. Put your left brain to useful work

As well as resting and disengaging the left brain, you can put it to work for you. You know that the left brain is good at logical analytical thought, so give it specific tasks to do.

Reduce the problem to its parts.

Identify which parts you have a measure of control over.

Work out specific strategies for those parts.

As an example, I once saw a man whose ex-wife was trying to gain custody of their two children. This man, David, was still reeling from the unexpected separation five months previously. Now his wife wanted to move interstate and take the children.

David was going crazy trying to work out why this had all happened and how he might fix it. However, the problem wasn't linear or logical, so left-brain thinking couldn't fix the whole thing. It could only help with the parts.

When he reduced the problem to smaller parts, he came up with two main issues. The first was that he couldn't work out why his wife had left him. The second was that he wanted his children to remain near him and he wanted joint custody.

The first of these two problems was clearly not at all logical and he would never find a black and white answer to his question. This type of thinking sends us crazy. For the moment, the logical thing to do was to concentrate on the other issue.

The left brain is much better at working out how David might get joint custody, or at least how to maximise his chances. So we reduce it further. Can he look after them financially? Does he have good legal advice? Will his work situation allow him to care for them appropriately? Does he have a house for them to live in? What reasons would his wife give to stop him getting joint custody and how would he counter these?

David then had a job for his left brain to do, working out strategies for each part of the problem. His other problem of why his wife left him is more complex but may have some logical components to it. The things his wife repeatedly said to him are useful to look at. 'You're never emotionally available,' or 'You work too hard,' or 'You don't pay attention to the children.' David may well learn a lot from the experience if he pays attention, but it is unlikely at this stage that he can change the outcome and get his wife back. To move forward he has to let go of that outcome.

5. Stop judging yourself

You know the left brain likes to classify things as good or bad, right or wrong, and because you are so attached to your left-brain way of thinking you always fall for this. You may think 'I am bad for thinking this thought or feeling this feeling.' Positive thinking strategies encourage you to replace such negative thoughts with their opposite positive ones. 'I am a good person.'

I suggest you try to stop judging yourself at all (and other people too). You just are – not good or bad, right or wrong – you just are. I just am. He just is. She just is.

The left brain loves to judge but you can stop this habit. All you have to do is live. In a holistic world, right and wrong don't exist in the way you have been led to believe. So when you catch your left brain judging yourself (or other people), try to let it go. It is just your left brain trying to classify the world the only way it knows how to (dualistically). Practise accepting yourself just as you are now. You can always change later.

6. Begin to use your other resources

As you stop relying on your left brain so much, you can begin to use your other resources.

You pay more attention to your right brain, your intuition and your feelings. You try to work out what your physical body is trying to tell you. You pay attention to the ether. You always try to go with the flow of the process of your life instead of battling against it. The following chapters outline how to take advantage of these other elements.

TWO - EARTH

Earth is the symbol of our physical presence. When we look at the planet earth, we see it is made up of a solid sphere of water and earth. This is surrounded by air and there is fire coming from the sun. The element earth is not the same as the planet earth. The element earth is the most solid of the elements, the most clearly 'matter', especially when compared to fire, which is more like spirit. The element earth is about our physical being.

Earth is soil, rock, mud, sand. It is solid and tangible. It changes slowly from one form to another, in contrast to water that changes more quickly. Earth is yin in nature – dark, receptive, mysterious. It gets its energy from the sun but it provides the nourishment for plants to grow, and therefore for animals to survive. It is sustaining. Earth provides the structure from which the rest of the system emerges. Plants grow towards the light (fire) and they need air and water to do this, but without the solid foundation of earth from which they draw their nourishment and anchor themselves, they have trouble surviving.

It is the same with humans. Our basic structure from which all else arises is our physical body. We may have all the ideas in the world and all the passions but without the basic health of our body to support these aspects, we will not flourish. We may be exceedingly spiritual people but to be whole we have to get our roots deep into the earth. We have to grow down as well as up.

We need to learn how best to nourish our own self.

At the most basic level, this involves a good diet, exercise and rest. For each of us this is an individual thing. Some of us need more sleep than others do. We all have different dietary needs. We have different requirements and capacities for exercise and activity. Yet we try to come up with a list of rules for diet and exercise that fits everyone. As individuals, we need to learn how to look after the physical body that we have been given. We need to learn what food suits us best, what exercises and activities enable us to be healthy, how much sleep we need.

On another level, we need to learn how to nourish our emotional self. We need to learn how to experience our feelings and learn what they mean for us.

We also need to learn how to nurture the connections between us and other people, how to connect with the planet earth in the most useful way, how to live in the community in a way that fulfils our individual needs as well as those of the community.

On another level, we need to nourish our air – our rational thinking brain and our intuitive brain. We do this by stimulating it and using it in ways that are meaningful to us as individuals.

We also need to nourish our fire. We need to nourish our passions and creativity and embrace our intuition.

As well as looking after our own nourishment, we need to pay some attention to nourishing the system that we are a part of. First, this means helping our friends and families nourish themselves. It means helping nourish the community we are a part of. It means helping to nourish the earth, especially in our immediate vicinity but also further afield. It means being aware that we are part of a larger system and therefore we help to look after the whole system.

Life is about balancing all our needs, the needs of those around us and those of the greater system. This is tricky because often the needs seem to be competing and we feel pulled in all sorts of directions, trying to be all things to all people. We may become selfish for a time and need to learn how to nurture ourselves so we can provide some nurturing of others and the earth.

The element earth – our physical body – is very good at letting us know about our needs but most of us do not pay it enough attention. So we get confused. If we begin to pay attention to ourselves, we start to understand what we need in order to live a whole life. What we need is unique to us.

Our inner self speaks to us through our physical body, letting us know what we need on an individual level. Every symptom we have, each disease we get, has a meaning. Sometimes the meaning is very physical – we are eating the wrong foods, not getting enough rest, working too hard. Sometimes the meaning is less easy to understand. However, the basis of all illness is this inner meaning about how we are not meeting our own needs. We may be compromising our self in ways that are not healthy, trying to be someone we are not, or we may just have things to learn from our illness that we can learn no other way.

Beliefs

Our ego has developed a set of beliefs based upon our upbringing. This set of beliefs arises from our families, our society, our friends, and all our influences.

We think that our belief system, that our collection of beliefs about how the world works, is truth. We believe that our beliefs are truth, when they are only beliefs about truth.

We might believe for instance that to be a spiritual person we should be nice to people. We think this is a spiritual truth when it is just a belief we hold in our heads. We might believe that we are a good teacher and a good parent and that those roles are what we should concentrate on. We believe this is who we are, when it is just a belief about who we are.

We have a huge collection of beliefs stored away, all of which are not how the world works but only beliefs about how the world works. Many of our beliefs are contradictory. Part of us might believe we are loveable while another part believes we are unlovable.

Most of us don't acknowledge the presence of these beliefs. We are not even conscious we have them. However, these beliefs often stand between who we think we are and who we really are, so our inner self is always trying to challenge them.

One of the ways soul brings these beliefs to our notice is through our physical body. The message from our soul via the body is always directed at how we can become ourselves, how we can be the person we are meant to be. Not the person society thinks we should be, not the person our friends and family expect us to be, not the person our left brain and ego tell us that we should be. The person we really are underneath all the beliefs about who we should be.

Our symptoms and our diseases have a greater meaning than we believe, but usually we have to discover this meaning for ourselves.

Within our illness lie the seeds of health.

My left brain had resisted this idea because it is so irrational and completely against everything I ever learnt as a doctor. Nevertheless, it is at the heart of this whole book. I began to see a different view and I continue to see different ways of being. Illness and disease have a literal meaning and a metaphorical meaning, a physical meaning and a spiritual or metaphysical meaning.

Patients are always teaching me how to be a better doctor. They share their stories and their lives with me in a way I never thought possible when I was at medical school. They sometimes bare their souls to me and it is at these times that I glimpse the wholeness and interconnectedness of us all.

I recently experienced a day in general practice like any other. I never know what to expect or where I will be led. I cannot remember all the patients I saw that day, but I remember two because they taught me more about the meaning behind our illnesses. They bared their souls so that I might see something extraordinary. They gave me a glimpse of their authentic inner selves fighting to be free of the person they had become.

The first woman I shall call Ruth. I have seen her as a patient over a number of years and she has had chronic fatigue syndrome for many years. She lives with it daily. I have talked to her in the past about how stress and her life are playing a part in this but for many reasons, I couldn't get her to see beyond her physical symptoms. Ruth came in at her wit's end, suicidal and depressed. Life was not worth living, she could see no hope that life would ever get any better. She asked me whether we should increase her medication.

For years, her chronic fatigue had been a way of her not being everything for everyone else, a way of her having some time out. It didn't really give her the time out her soul needed because she was always fighting against the belief that she might put herself ahead of everyone else's needs. Ruth told me that she had always been this way in order to please others and to be loved. Now she felt that if she was loved it wasn't for who she really was but for what she did for others. She was having trouble seeing who she really was.

She had spent her whole life pleasing and helping other people because she believed that this was how to show love to her family. She believed that to be a good person she should put everyone else's needs before her own. Now, her inner self was telling her that she needed time out to discover who she really was. She needed to find out who the real Ruth was.

I didn't have to tell Ruth this, she told me. This is the only way we really discover the meaning behind our illness – we have to discover it ourselves. It's as if suddenly we understand why our life has become the way it is and how we might move forward to change it. We may see numerous health professionals who might lead us towards a better understanding, but until we 'get it' ourselves we cannot move on. This 'getting it' is a function of our right brain and often comes when we realise we can't rationally solve the problem, nor can the many doctors we have seen.

Ruth began by telling me her life wasn't worth living and that she might as well die. She progressed to tell me that this particular life wasn't worth living; it wasn't the life she needed. She told me that she could sleep for twelve months, she felt like packing her bags and leaving, she needed space to find out who she was.

I felt privileged to be present at her moment of self-discovery. All I did was to be open enough to hear the message from her inner self. I considered changing her medication in an attempt to alleviate the symptoms but I knew this was just a Band-Aid measure and it probably wouldn't even work. My intuition knew that Ruth needed to talk and all I needed to do was listen. By hearing the meaning beneath the story, Ruth could hear that meaning too.

Ruth's story hadn't really changed but suddenly she could hear the deeper meanings for herself. One of the ways we heal ourselves is by understanding the messages inherent in the story of our life.

What healers do is to help their patients pay attention to their own messages, help them learn more about themselves and how they can heal.

Ruth helped me learn that what I am writing about works, that diseases and circumstances always have messages for us. If we listen to the message and listen to our inner selves, we will be able to find our own answers.

At the end of the consultation, my doctor's left brain wanted to take back a little control but Ruth simply said, 'I know where to go from here, I just have to look inside and decide what I want to believe in.'

I had done nothing except be present. Being present for another person is a powerful way we can help others.

The next patient, Norma, was one who I had seen earlier that morning with chest pain, abdominal pain, tiredness, pain in the neck, and social problems. I had sent her off for some tests, she had returned to the surgery, and she had been waiting a while to see me. I was already late for lunch.

I am trying to practise what I preach in this book but part of me is still firmly a medical doctor, with all that that implies. When I allow my inner self rather than my ego to run the show, things always go better, but they often take longer. Listening to people's inner self is difficult to do in fifteen minutes. Norma sat in front of me with her ECG. My rational doctor part wanted to deal with that and have lunch. My inner self, however, had just been doing its thing with the previous patient and wasn't ready to give up on this one.

I can't remember how we got to it but within minutes, Norma was telling me that she felt as if she was always doing everything for everyone else and that she didn't know who she really was.

I had a moment of déjà vu and felt that something powerful and wonderful was happening. I was in the middle of writing a book about how to get in touch with who you really are and here were two women telling me the same things I was writing about. This felt weird but one of the things I have learnt about spirit is that if things feel weird then powerful forces are at work.

Norma and I talked about much the same things that Ruth and I had talked about. She told me she needed space to work out who she was, away from the everyday demands of her family. She told me that much of what she did was in response to the voice in her head telling her that she should behave the way she had been, but it wasn't really who she was. Back in 'doctor, it's time for lunch' mode, I told her she should stop looking after everyone else and start looking after herself. She told me that it wasn't time yet but that when certain things happened and certain obligations had been fulfilled it would be time.

You might ask what all this has to do with symptoms and diseases being messages. For Ruth, her chronic disease had been sending her a message for years that she was living under a set of rules and beliefs that weren't useful for her. She was discovering that she needed to find herself rather than be someone who everyone else (and up to this point her ego) expected her to be. It had taken her many years to understand the message finally, partly because the medical system had never looked at it in this way either.

For Norma, the individual symptoms could have individual messages but the whole lot of them told her that her body was reacting to the stress in her life. We had started out looking for causes and ended up talking about how she needed to find who she really was. She told me the symptoms were her body's way of telling her to look after herself instead of everyone else. She already knew that deep inside.

Both women went away with their own answers. I had not given them these answers; they had been inside of them all along. I had just been able to keep my own ego out of the way long enough for them to step aside from theirs and glimpse their inner selves. They had been searching for a connection with their inner self, which had been trying to reach them through the messages inherent in their symptoms and diseases.

Our inner selves give us symptoms and diseases so that we may become the person we are meant to be. Not the person the rest of the world and our ego wish us to be, but the person deep inside struggling to get out. These symptoms and diseases are gifts. Of course, we don't see them as gifts. We see them as restrictions and obstacles to our life. We see them as problems to be overcome so that we can get back to the life we were leading before these troublesome symptoms got in the way. We see these diseases as chaos.

This is the gift from our soul. Within each disease lie the seeds of health.

An egocentric, physically orientated life is not the one our inner self seeks. If an illness is preventing us from living that life, it is doing a good job. If we treat the symptoms and the illness and return to the life we were leading, we have failed to receive the gift in the spirit that it was intended. The message is always to change something about our world. We may need to change something about what we believe, or we may need to change some of our behaviours. We may need to access parts of ourselves that we have previously been unconscious of.

None of this is simple. There are always layers and complications so that no health care provider or expert can give you a simple answer to your health problem. If they do, it is likely the answers are only at one level, often superficial. The answers we are all looking for are available if we look deeper.

Our culture and our health care system concentrate on the superficial. If we have a health problem, we want to fix it with a tablet or some other quick solution. We don't want to be bothered with working out why we have the problem and what we can do to fix it ourselves. We have been led to believe that we can't take responsibility for our own health and that we need experts to fix everything.

We need to learn that most of our health problems can be fixed by listening to our inner self. Most of us have forgotten how to do this. I see many patients who, against their intuition, undergo invasive investigations, surgeries and drug treatments that often result in more illness.

Modern medicine has an important place, but it is not the answer to all our health issues. Modern medicine often uses superficial solutions that usually do nothing to heal our deeper problems, which are always related to disconnection from our wholeness.

To find the deeper meaning behind our illness, we need to stop trying to solve the problem of illness in a purely rational manner and look instead at what the lessons are.

Four ways to help your physical body

1. Treat your body well

A common problem within our society is our disregard for our human body. We sometimes forget that we are here in physical form. We do this because we believe that our minds are who we really are, or because we believe ourselves to be spiritual beings who really don't need a body. Whatever the many and varied reasons behind this, we often find ourselves disconnected from our physicality.

We forget that we are partly earth, that our presence on earth is physical for many reasons and that one of our tasks here is to manifest our inner self through our physical being.

Our body often reminds us of this. It reminds us that how we treat it affects it – this is often a linear effect. We drink too much alcohol, and we feel sick. We exercise too little and eat too much, and we get fat. We drive too fast, and we hit a tree and are injured. The laws of the physical world affect our physical bodies and we can't ignore them. (We might be able to train ourselves to subvert these physical laws – yogis and other people can do so – but largely our physical bodies are bound by physical laws.)

Often our illness and physical symptoms are direct reminders that our bodies cannot do everything we want. We all have limits. Illness provides a means of grounding ourselves, of bringing ourselves back to earth. When we have a bad case of the flu or if we injure our back, we suddenly have to pay attention to the fact that we have a body and it's not doing what we want it to. We have to become more grounded, more in tune with our body.

We may have been working too hard, not sleeping enough, eating too much junk, and abusing our body in any number of ways. We probably didn't pay attention to the small messages – the tiredness, lack of energy, grumpiness – we just carried on as if we were superheros with no limits. 'Suddenly', we find ourselves flat on our backs. We might lie there frustrated and angry with our bodies. Or we might lie there contemplating life and the ways in which we forgot that we were human.

We can avoid much of our illness if we treat our body well. Sleep when we are tired. Eat when we are hungry. Do what feels right, what makes us feel good physically, and pay more attention to what doesn't feel right.

2. Pay attention to your body

One reason we don't treat our body well is because we have forgotten to pay it attention. Our body will let us know when what we are doing is not what we need to do. In holistic medicine, the physical is a reflection of the spiritual, and vice-versa. If we neglect our physical body, we are also neglecting our inner self. There are, however, no specific rules for how you should treat your body because everyone is different. What we all need to do is learn how to treat our own body well. What we eat, how we exercise, how much sleep we need is individual. Everything is individual and we need to pay enough attention so that we can work out what we need.

If your body doesn't feel well then you probably aren't treating it well. We can all try to follow the latest fad diet or use the latest miracle antioxidant cure. However, until we start to pay attention to how our body is reacting to everything we put in it and do to it, then we won't be able to learn what we, as an individual, need to do to be our best physically.

I have discovered in my own life that I am at my best when I sleep at least eight hours a night, walk regularly, eat a mostly vegetarian diet, and don't work too hard. I have discovered that my body does not do well on fasts, that I need regular amounts of food to feel good. I have discovered that I need a certain amount of alone time to feel my best but that I also need time with friends and family. I have discovered that I need to nurture my connection with the earth by gardening and walking in the bush and being near the sea. I have learnt that I need to link myself into my community in ways that are fulfilling for me. I have learnt that I need to honour my passions and my creativity but balance this by being grounded. I have learnt many things about myself and I am still learning. I find out all these things not by referring to some expert who tells me how to live, but by always referring back to myself and to what is happening in my life.

Paying attention is about paying attention to the literal – if you are tired you need more sleep, if you are overweight you are eating too much or doing too little, if you have a sore knee you may have been doing too much with it. But it is also about paying attention to the deeper meanings. Sometimes we are tired because we are doing too many things that we really don't need to do. Sometimes we are overweight because we are hiding our true self behind layers of insulation. Sometimes our knee hurts because we are going the wrong direction in life.

In paying attention to our body's messages, we need to pay attention on both a physical and a spiritual level. So we look at the literal meaning behind our disease and also at the metaphorical (or spiritual) meaning.

3. Learn to translate the body's messages

The body's messages can be literal and physical or they can be metaphorical and spiritual. Most of us can begin to understand the literal physical meaning just by thinking about it or consulting a conventional health practitioner. But with the literal meanings, always remember that you are an individual and that you need to work out for yourself what you need. You might begin with general rules or guidelines but you need to refine them for yourself.

Metaphorical or spiritual meanings of physical symptoms are not something most of us are used to, but they reflect our inner needs. A problem with our eyes may reflect an inability to see something about ourselves or about our lives. A hoarse voice may reflect a problem we have with saying something that is difficult for us to say. A problem with our leg may indicate an issue we have about the direction our life is heading.

The best books I have found to help with symptom interpretation are The Body is the Barometer of the Soul by Annette Noontil, The Secret Language of your Body by Inna Segal and Your Body's Telling you: Love Yourself by Lise Bourbeau.[12] Louise Hay has also written extensively on this subject.

These books are, however, just tools to enable you to find a deeper meaning in your symptoms or diseases. They will give you an idea of what your inner self may be trying to tell you but as always, they are not to be taken as truth. Sometimes your symptoms and illnesses will have other meanings that only you can decipher. Sometimes they will have multiple meanings and you will only discover them as you live the process of your life and the illness. When we have as an outcome the idea that we can cure our illnesses, we forget that sometimes our illnesses are part of longer-term lessons that we can only learn from living with the illness.

As an example, someone I know developed type 1 diabetes in his thirties. The books give various meanings for this but it is my belief that this person needed the diabetes over many years in order to learn how to look after his physical body better. This person has a tendency to prefer to live in the spiritual realms. His diabetes means that his conscious attention is always being brought back to his physical body. In this way, his inner self is continually reminding him that he is human.

12   Publishing details in the Bibliography.

Many of our illnesses bring us back to the basics of life. Often we forget what is important to us as individuals and suddenly we find we are living a life that is not what we need. Illness often plays a part in helping us realise this. We always have to take stock and prune back the parts of our life that we no longer need. Some of us have chronic illness because we don't pay some part of ourselves enough attention. We believe we are superhuman or gods. The only way for our inner self to demonstrate the error in this thinking is to give us an illness.

4. Earthing or grounding ourselves

When we are ill, it is usually because some part of us needs to be more grounded and connected to the earth – or to the people of the earth, that is, family and community. In this way, illness brings our focus back to the essentials. We are flat on our back reliant upon others to help look after us.

Illness always brings us back to earth – that is why we dislike it so much. It limits us and makes us feel that we cannot do what we want to do. We are forced to connect more with the earth and with the people of the earth. This happens because most of us are too full of air and fire. We may consciously become more aware of this and consciously earth ourselves.

Grounding helps us re-establish our connection to the earth. Grounding activities, such as exercise, gardening, walking barefoot along the beach, are activities that matter to a physical being. They remind us that we live in a physical world and inhabit physical, and therefore mortal, bodies. We can always take time out to ground ourselves better by doing physical things, which put us in touch with our body.

We can deliberately ground ourselves in times of inner or outer turmoil by increasing our connection to the earth. To do this, sit, stand or lie on the earth and sink into it. Feel the earth beneath you and feel the connection between you and the earth. Tune into the areas where your body connects with the earth and visualise or feel this connection increasing. Feel yourself solidly connected with the earth.

By grounding ourselves, we increase our connection to the earth and we increase our awareness of the needs of the earth. We are all part of the larger system that is earth and one of our needs is to nurture the system that we are part of. We can do this by paying attention to how we live and realising that the earth is a finite thing. The resources of the earth cannot be used up without endangering the whole system. We begin to pay attention to how we live on the earth and whether we are taking more from her than we really need. We begin to think not only about ourselves but also about the whole system.

Connecting ourselves with other people means that we find our place in our family and community, and nurture this. We become connected by giving and taking. We give what we need to give and we receive what we need. Most of us are unbalanced in this regard. The imbalance is not as simple as giving more than we can and taking less than we need, or taking more than we need and giving less than we can. Most of us are so out of touch with what we really need that we never get our needs met. We are so out of touch with what others need from us that we have no idea how to help others.

I will discuss this more in the chapter on ether, but we all need to learn how to get our own needs met and how to help others meet their needs. The simplest thing we need to learn is the difference between what we want and what we need. Most of us have too much of what we think we want and too little of what we really need.

Connecting with other people means identifying some of our needs and asking other people to meet them. It also means identifying what other people in our families and communities need and working out how we can play our part in meeting those needs.

THREE - WATER

Water is the element of feeling and emotions. We have learnt to treat feelings as if they are thoughts. We have learnt to try to control them. This is not what they are about.

Feelings are like water – they can sit like deep pools or they can flow and cycle. We do best when we allow them to do what water does naturally, to cycle and flow. Even deep pools evaporate and become rain and fall somewhere else. The properties of cycling and flowing enable us to see how we might experience our feelings better.

Water is essentially yin. This means that our feelings are a way of receiving information about ourselves, about our needs and about the needs of those around us. The yang aspect of feelings is that sometimes when we ignore their messages, they will erupt with great force and we will act on them (sometimes in ways we don't like!). This happens most when we refuse to acknowledge their presence. We do this because we have been taught that it is inappropriate to have certain feelings.

In Western society, we are generally taught that it is inappropriate to feel so-called 'bad' feelings – anger, hate, bitterness – so we learn how not to feel them.

When we allow ourselves to feel the anger or the frustration, we undergo a process of growth. A feeling state helps us to work through something that is going on in our lives, allowing us to move forward. We move closer to our own self and therefore are closer to being whole. We do not do this by thinking about the feelings or talking about the feelings, rather we do it by feeling the feelings and allowing them to take us to a different place. We allow the meaning to reveal itself.

We have learnt five main ways of controlling our feelings.[13]

1. Denial

When we are in denial, we bury our feelings and cover them up. We put our feelings away from our consciousness and pretend they don't exist.

Most of us use denial at some stage in our lives. We usually don't even realise we are using it, because we have removed the experience of our feelings from our conscious awareness.

Denial is a useful technique for our ego when it doesn't want to face something. This might help us in times of crisis when so many things are changing that we can't cope unless we pretend things haven't changed. When someone dies unexpectedly, our immediate response is, 'No, that can't be'. This is denial at work. While denial like all our ego defences is useful at times, when we use it all the time we run into trouble.

Ego defences such as denial are subconscious. We don't consciously deny that something has happened or deny that we are feeling something, we put it away from our conscious mind. We don't know in our thinking brain that we have denied it. Our thinking brain actually believes that it is true. When I use denial in order not to feel something, my thinking brain actually believes I am not feeling it.

---

13   There are other ways that people avoid feelings, which you might know or discover, but these five are the main ones people use.

How can we know we are using denial? Obviously, it is tricky because it is such an unconscious process. We therefore need to pay close attention to our other elements. Is our intuition talking to us? For example, are we having dreams that might let us know? Is our body sending us a message – do our symptoms tell us about a feeling? Is our thinking trying to tell us anything – are we obsessing about an issue? Are there any signs from the universe – is someone telling us that we are a hard-hearted person? Sometimes denial is used because we aren't quite ready to face our feelings. Eventually they will surface.

When we use denial all the time, we effectively shut ourselves off from one of our inner aspects. Generally, feelings cannot be contained forever so when they erupt they may erupt with great power. When we use denial a lot, we put ourselves at risk of depression and serious health problems.

2. Rationalisation

If you listen to your left brain, you will hear it rationalising all the time. 'I shouldn't feel like this', 'no-one else feels like this', 'I won't feel this'.

Some of these rationalisations are useful but some of them avoid feelings.

I shouldn't feel so sad about my dog dying; it's only a dog after all.

I shouldn't feel angry at Barry for not buying me a birthday present.

I shouldn't feel in love with Sheryl because she doesn't love me.

I shouldn't feel anxious about the job interview.

I shouldn't feel scared about abseiling.

All of these are rationalisations.

We often convince ourselves that we don't feel something because our brain tells us we shouldn't. Our brain only tells us that because of our belief that this is so. The feeling will not simply go away because our brain tells us it shouldn't be there. By suppressing a feeling, we contain the feeling. Feelings have meaning. Until we feel them and discover the meaning, rationalising won't get rid of them.

Sometimes we encourage rationalisation by talking about our feelings too much. Although talking about our feelings may help us recognise them, if we talk about them in an analytical way we have started the rationalisation process. When we pull apart and dissect our feelings, we fall into the trap of believing they are like thoughts. The power of feelings is in their flow, so we often never reach a rational understanding of them. This is another case of thinking too much.

We need to discover the meaning behind the feeling, and this is usually an intuitive process. Often we want to know why we are feeling something – what is the cause? This is part of the rationalisation, part of our left brain trying to pull apart something that cannot be understood in this way.

3. Lost in translation

When we let our ego beliefs translate a feeling into an emotional state, our pure feelings become mixed emotional messages instead. They become contaminated and difficult to understand.

We may feel fear but ego translates it to anger. When our child falls off the swing and gets hurt, the deeper feelings of love and fear for the loved one are translated into anger. Instead of projecting love, we project anger and yell at the child for being silly.

We may feel love for someone but ego translates part of the love as anxiety. The anxiety comes from our fear of rejection so instead of projecting love onto our loved one, we project anxiety and fear of rejection.

When someone we love dies, we feel sad but often ego translates this into anger – we have to blame someone or something for the death in order not to feel our sadness.

If we reflect on our feelings, we can start to translate them back into the pure feeling. If I feel angry with someone I might ask myself, is that anger really towards myself? What deeper feeling might my anger be masking? Usually just being open to the feeling and sitting with it allows the feeling to transform into what it is really about.

4. Acting out

We act out our feelings, often on other people. We may become violent, act like victims, become passive or aggressive. When we act out our feelings, we are really acting out our pain. We don't allow ourselves to own the feeling and instead, project it onto other people. We delude ourselves that they have a problem rather than it being our own problem.

Once we allow our feelings to move through us without needing to project them onto other people, we are more able to control our actions. If we can be open to our anger and own it as our anger rather than coming from someone else, we begin to own our actions. Instead of lashing out at someone we love when we begin to get angry, we open ourselves up to the feeling of anger and pay attention to where it takes us. It is not about acting in any way we like and blaming it on our anger. It is about opening ourselves to the feeling and resisting the urge to act it out until we understand its message.

When we let ourselves feel anger, we often realise why we are angry and then we can take steps to do something about the situation that has produced our anger. This is where logic and rational thought may help us sort out the best action but first, we need to acknowledge the feeling.

5. Avoidance

We develop ways to avoid our feelings by replacing them with addictions or by filling up our lives with so much stuff that we have no room to feel.

Most of us avoid feelings by never giving ourselves space or time to feel them. A friend of mine lost his wife and went back to work the next week. He said if he kept busy, he didn't have to feel as much. All of us use this tactic and sometimes it may be useful. My friend was overwhelmed by his feelings and needed time out from them. His work helped provide that time out. But when we do this all the time, we have a problem.

When our lives are so busy and full that we have no time to think, we have to realise we also have no time to feel. Feelings need time. They need to be able to filter into our consciousness and they can only do that if we give them space.

If you have trouble sitting still, if the thought of a quiet night at home by yourself fills you with dread, if your life is always full of people and things and you never get a minute to yourself, then it is likely that you are using all those things to avoid facing your own feelings.

The other way we avoid our feelings is by taking something like alcohol, prescription drugs or illegal drugs. Often, we do this in combination with denial. Sometimes we become addicted to work or food or exercise to avoid feeling.

Most of us choose one or two of these ways preferentially. If we look at ourselves truthfully, we usually see which ways we prefer to use. We are all capable of using any of these methods to avoid feeling.

We avoid feeling not only because society teaches us that we should, but because we believe that feelings are too painful and a sign of weakness. We believe that some feelings are good and others are bad and that we should only feel good feelings. We believe that anger is bad and that we shouldn't feel it, or that sadness is a weakness, or that happiness must be earned.

All of these are beliefs, not truth.

Too little water

If you are not paying attention to your feelings, it's like wearing a blindfold or pretending you are blind. Not to use one of your senses when you have the opportunity is really pretty silly. If you think it makes no difference to your life, try walking around with a blindfold for a day. That is what many of us are doing when we don't take full advantage of our feelings. Feelings are not a liability; they are an evolutionary advantage that we often fail to make the most of.

If we avoid our feelings, we put ourselves at greater risk of illness. Blindfolding ourselves puts us at risk of injury – we end up walking into doors and tables. Metaphorically blindfolding our feelings puts us at greater risk of many illnesses, including heart attacks and depression.

How do we remove the blindfold?

We do so by deciding that we want to. Like any habit, we need to remember that we won't let it go easily. We will be full of good intentions but unless we continually practise seeing the world without our blindfold, we will have trouble. Every time we take off our blindfold, the light will hurt our eyes and we will be tempted to shut our eyes from the glare. As we become accustomed to the light, it will become easier.

So we take off our blindfold. Then we look at it closely. Is it mainly a blindfold of denial or rationalisation, of emotional overreaction or of acting out? Is our blindfold made up of all these strands?

By identifying how we blindfold our feelings, we can work out how we might stop doing so. We have to catch ourselves every time we try to put the blindfold on.

When we hear our ego voice rationalising something, we wonder if we are rationalising away an emotion and then pay attention to how we are really feeling.

When we feel ourselves getting angry and out of control, we step back and pay attention to how we feel deep inside.

When we get emotional and overwhelmed, we look inside and wonder whether we are avoiding a deeper issue.

When we notice we eat or drink alcohol or take drugs to avoid feeling, we pay attention to this. We don't bother blaming ourselves for using any of these defences against our feelings because we realise change is a process.

We have taken off our blindfold.

We examine it and start paying attention to when we try to put it back on.

We look inside and try to feel our feelings. We let our feelings wash over us like water and see where they take us. Sometimes the message they bring is clear, at other times it makes no sense. Each time we start to trust that our feelings have a meaning and a place in our lives, we let go of ego control a little more.

Love is the feeling we all wish we had more of and our feelings try to take us to a deeper understanding of love. But we often find the process too painful so we avoid it.

The choice is in whether we open our hearts or close them. We can choose whether to embrace our soul and its spirit, or our ego and its defences. Although we might try to deny we have a choice, we know we do by the feelings we experience.

When my friend Angela died, there was a pain in my chest that wouldn't go away. My choice was to embrace the pain and open my heart to it, or keep my heart closed and try to deny the pain. I chose the latter because I hadn't even considered the former a possibility.

I got angry, I wanted to blame someone, I wanted an answer to why she had died, I felt that life wasn't fair. For a while, I raged against the changes that her death brought. But gradually my soul let me know that these ways of thinking were just making things worse. There was no-one to blame or get angry at. There was no reason why she died. Life simply isn't fair in a left-brained way.

Without even realising I had a choice, I began to open my heart a little and let the process of grieving have its way with me. I did nothing for the first week except let myself grieve as I needed to. After that, life crowded in on me but still I allowed time just to 'be' with the feelings. I let them wash over me, let the tears flow and the anger erupt if I needed to.

As time went on the flow of my feelings eased the pain. In opening my heart, I opened it to all the love that still existed in my life. Angela and I had never said we loved each other, it just wasn't that sort of friendship, but in many ways I wished I had been able to express the feelings to her while she was alive. Then I had a vivid dream. It involved a familiar scene at her house. As I was leaving, she usually came outside with me to see me off but this time she stayed inside. As I got to my car I realised I needed to say goodbye so I went back inside. As I went back through the door, Angela was standing at the end of the entrance as if waiting for me. We gave each other a big hug, she told me she loved me, I told her I loved her, and then we said goodbye.

I woke up feeling that she had returned to do this for me, as if her spirit had crept into my dream to say goodbye and express the love between us. I don't know if this would have happened so quickly if I had continued suppressing and denying my feelings.

I am continually learning about my own resistance to 'being' with my feelings. I was very upset at a friend of mine recently but I wasn't sure what to do about it. Eventually I told him that I was upset by something he had done. He asked me if I was angry.

Of course I was angry but I immediately rationalised it all away and tried to pretend that I wasn't feeling anger. I did this largely because I have learnt that I shouldn't get angry with people. My brain tells me, 'Don't get angry with people you love.' Actually it goes a step beyond that and tells me, 'Don't even *feel* angry with people you love; even feeling anger is not right.'

What I now choose to believe is that feeling anger is okay. I don't have to show or tell the other person that I am angry, and I don't have to act out my anger. But I do have to feel it.

I went outside by myself to feel my anger. I let myself be angry. I yelled and paced and shook my fists. I did this for about half an hour, and gradually the anger that I thought was about my friend became about me.

My anger was telling me that I was acting in a way that wasn't meeting my needs, that I wasn't being myself.

There was not a linear connection between the anger and the realisation, but there was a connection. By letting myself feel the anger, it showed me something very important about myself, about how I was interacting with my friend. It showed me that I needed to do something about the situation. Usually, I find anger is about my inability to say no to other people's demands on me. That was what happened with my friend. I can only get rid of the anger when I begin to put my own needs ahead of everyone else's.

Following the process of our feelings is a useful way to uncover their messages. This means 'being' with the feelings rather than avoiding them. When we feel something, we need to go inward to discover the message. The message from our feelings is not a message from our external world but a message from our internal world telling us that something is happening.

What is happening, if we allow it, is that our feelings are taking us to a deeper understanding of ourselves and the ways in which we might grow.

Too much water

When we don't pay attention to our feelings, when we don't let them flow through us and around us, we risk the 'deep well' syndrome. Water can stand in deep wells for long periods, just as feelings can lie within us for long periods. When we don't feel them and follow their meaning, we risk sending them deep into our unconscious. We end up with a pool of feelings that we have never dealt with but that constantly affects us, yet we have no idea why we are affected.

This deep well of feelings that we have never connected with threatens to drown us at certain times in our lives. When new intense feelings begin to arise at times of crisis or stress, we become overwhelmed with the deepness of the well. The new feelings bring the well of old feelings to our awareness and it can be a mighty deep and scary well, full of dark unknown fears.

Some of us block ourselves off from the well by attempting to feel nothing – this leads to depression. Some of us get scared by the depth of the well, leading to anxiety symptoms. Some of us experience physical symptoms.

This deep well syndrome often arises from childhood traumas or from very traumatic experiences in our past. Many of us are ill equipped to deal with it because we have never learnt how to feel properly.

Many types of counselling and therapy can help empty this deep well, but the best way to empty it is to begin to practise feeling. As we learn how to feel the whole range of feelings, we can begin to let go of past feelings and find a way to meet our needs. As with all things, we are individuals and so we will find what we need to help us empty our well. We may need counselling, psychotherapy or some physical treatments. As we begin to pay better attention to our feelings (all of them), we learn more about getting our needs met and helping other people meet theirs.

We all have deep wells of emotion and for most of us, they are connected to learned patterns of behaviour. We continually repeat some patterns of behaviour because this is how we learnt to cope with certain feelings. When a feeling is triggered, the pattern of behaviour follows. Such patterns of behaviour belong in the past where they were once useful. We need to shed old patterns of behaviour that are no longer useful. I will discuss this more in Part four.

Five Ways to Feel Better

1. Honesty

We would all like to believe that we are honest people. Yet all of us lie. We tell our biggest lies to ourselves. We tell ourselves we don't feel a certain way because we believe that if we have so-called 'bad' feelings, it makes us bad people. Feelings are often not politically correct. We can feel hate towards the people we love just as easily as we can towards our enemies. We feel jealousy and anger and sadness and we somehow believe this makes us morally bad.

Becoming honest with ourselves means being honest about how we feel. We don't need to act on the feelings or tell people about them, but in order to become whole people we need to learn how to feel them. This starts with acknowledging that they are present.

We are learning how to be more honest and this begins always with ourselves – becoming aware when we are lying to ourselves.

I might feel angry with my partner but I can choose what I do about the anger. When I am not being honest with myself, I tend to deny I have the anger but because feelings have energy, my partner will know something is wrong. He may deny it also so that we collude in ignoring my anger. The longer we ignore it the more it builds until one day, over some small irritation, it will burst out of me. I make a mountain out of a molehill because I have a mountain of unacknowledged anger inside me.

If I can be more honest with myself, I might just sit with the angry feelings and let them wash over me.

Feelings are like water. As I let myself shower in my angry feelings, the anger eventually flows away. Some other feeling or an insight into the situation replaces it. Once I have acknowledged the anger and let it be felt, then I am in a much better position to change something.

The feeling is my feeling not my partner's. Something about our interaction has triggered the anger. He has not caused me to feel the anger in a direct way, but something about our relationship has caused it. Usually I am angry because in some way I am not getting some of my needs met but until I let the anger come out, I am unable to discover its message.

If I cannot be honest with myself and admit that I feel angry, then the anger has nowhere to go but inside.

2. Accept the feelings

Stop judging feelings as good or bad and just accept that they are. Anger is not a bad feeling. It usually lets us know something about the situation we are in. It often tells us that we are not happy to be in this situation and tries to get us to move or to change the situation.

Commonly, anger arises because we are unable to ask for what we need yet we still expect to get it. When I get angry with my partner for not giving me enough space, it is usually because I am unable to ask for the space. Part of me has been led to believe that I shouldn't need space if I love someone, so I don't always recognise this need myself, until I get grumpy and angry. Then I recognise what is happening.

I might feel sad because I still miss Angela, so I accept this feeling and let myself cry and it passes.

Sometimes when I am really happy, I begin to get scared that this will mean at some stage I will have to feel sadness. Part of accepting feelings is to acknowledge that we will feel a range of feelings in our lives. When I connect deeply with people and feel the love between us, this makes me feel happy. But because I am human, there is a downside to this feeling. Any attachment to another person means that we will feel loss and sadness when they leave.

All we can be sure of is that feelings flow and pass. They never stay with us forever. Happiness is always transitory. Sadness is always transitory. Feelings teach us how to live in the now – live in the happiness and joy when it is here. They also teach us about hope and the future. When we feel at our worst, we can know that this too will pass.

3. Don't become the feeling

Feelings, like thoughts, are part of us but they are not us. We can try to separate ourselves from them and just observe them. When we do this, the feelings can pass through us and deliver their messages. Even good feelings can't be captured – they come and go.

Good feelings let us know that something we are doing is right for us. If something makes us happy, the message is partly to do more of this. We all need to have joy and happiness in our lives and the way to get more of this is to pay particular attention to what makes us happy and find ways in our life to cultivate those things. We always need to remember that what makes us happy today may not make us happy tomorrow. What makes us happy when we do it for an hour may not make us happy if we do it for ten.

I love to spend time with my family and friends so I try to make that a priority, but if I spend too much time with them, it no longer makes me happy. I need to balance it with my other needs, to have some time alone to think and write, to spend time alone with my partner, to spend time at work. I am happy being a mother and fulfilling some of my children's needs but I can't do that to the exclusion of my own needs. When I begin to get angry and frustrated, I step back and wonder how I am not getting my own needs met. Usually it is because I am doing too much for my children and not enough for myself.

A so-called negative feeling is usually a signal that we need to change something in our lives. We may need to change our beliefs, our expectations, our behaviours, or our circumstances.

4. Pay attention to the message and the meaning

Feelings have meaning for us as individuals and we need to pay enough attention to them in order to discover what that is.

Generally, the meaning behind good feelings is that what we are doing is making us feel good. We could do more of whatever that is. The meaning behind the not-so-good feelings is that what we are doing is in some way making us feel not so good. We need to do less of whatever that is.

This may seem simple but many of us have forgotten that we have a measure of control over our lives. We can choose to do more of what makes us feel good and less of what makes us feel not so good.

Sometimes with not-so-good feelings, we have trouble working out what is contributing to them. If we do not let our feelings 'be', then we have trouble interpreting them. Learning about feeling better is learning about how to feel all feelings. Once we feel the bad feelings, we learn to interpret their meanings. We can't come up with a list of what feelings mean because they are individual.

I once saw a woman who was engaged to be married. She came in with anxiety symptoms that were getting worse the closer she got to her wedding day. She had tried everything she knew to stop the anxiety attacks. I encouraged her to feel the anxiety. What was it about? Initially, she didn't know but then she identified that she got most anxious when she thought about the wedding or had to do some planning for it. I suggested that she was anxious about getting married. She tried to deny this because she thought she shouldn't feel anxious about getting married. I then encouraged her to stop judging the feeling as right or wrong, and accept and take more notice of it instead of trying to ignore it. She did this for a while and then realised that she wasn't sure that her fiancé was the right person to marry. She still felt a strong connection to her past boyfriend who she could talk to on a more intimate level about her feelings and needs, but who was totally unreliable. She felt torn between the reliable fiancé and the ex-boyfriend.

This woman then went through a tumultuous period. She called off her wedding and spent time talking to her fiancé about the anxiety and the issues that it brought up for her. She was able to talk to him about her needs and she ended up developing a deeper connection with her fiancé and deciding that she didn't really want to be with her ex-boyfriend after all. They put their wedding plans on hold but deepened their commitment to each other. The anxiety symptoms disappeared.

There was no simple answer behind the anxiety. It involved this woman being willing to feel it and discover her own meaning. This led her to a greater understanding of her own needs and an ability to talk to her partner about those needs.

Often, the interpretation of feelings is complex and requires that we follow the process of our lives until we discover the meaning for ourselves.

5. Enjoy the positive feelings

Sometimes we forget to enjoy enjoyable feelings. We may think that we don't deserve them or that they won't last. Because feelings act like water, they come and go but that doesn't mean we shouldn't enjoy them when they are here. We could take joy when we find it and bask in love. We could laugh and be happy as much as we possibly can. These positive feelings feed our soul and inner self. They give us energy to do what we need to do even when it is sometimes hard and not much fun.

FOUR - FIRE

Fire is the hardest of the four basic elements to categorise. Fire is very yang so it is a strong active element, but it isn't very solid. It's hard to grasp. Fire brings us new ideas and plans and the energy to carry them out. Fire is full of passion and action but it can also be full of destruction. A fire can warm us and make us feel good or it can burn out of control and destroy everything in its path. Like all our other elements, fire has a dual nature, the capacity to create and to destroy.

All the elements can be categorised into their yin and yang aspects. The yang side of fire is the active side – the creating, the action, the drive to create or destroy, the burning bright ideas that captivate others and encourage them to follow. The yin side is softer and less obvious. It is the receptive side, our intuitive ability, where ideas are received and nurtured. This side of fire is often forgotten or not nurtured. For fire to be balanced, it needs both parts. Receiving and nurturing and then acting.

Yin fire

Intuition is an internal sensing. We receive our intuitive messages through our physical body in ways related to our primary senses, usually the three main ones – sight, touch and hearing. We might see things (dreams, daydreams or visions), we might hear things (thoughts, voices, songs), or we might feel things (gut feelings, fear, anxiety). Some people have intuitive senses through taste and smell but these are less common.

All of us can learn to access our intuition better but some people are naturally good at it. The first step is always about learning how to trust our intuition as a reliable source of information. I will discuss this further later on in this chapter.

Yang fire

The yang aspect of fire is active. This is the creative (and destructive) fire. Yin fire without its yang aspect ends up doing nothing. None of the creative ideas and understandings can be physically manifested without the yang fire. The yin fire is the spark or the ember, the yang is the flame. The flame needs lots of air and earth (wood) to keep it going.

This is the part of us that manifests things in the physical world. This is why this element is sometimes likened to spirit. Fire is the underlying energy that drives us to create things physically; it allows us to manifest our essential spirit on earth.

Some new-age thinkers have taken this idea of manifestation and led people to believe that anyone is capable of manifesting anything. This is a linear view of manifestation and it isn't fully correct. We can all manifest things on a physical level but our particular fire determines what we manifest. We do not manifest things by simply thinking about them and believing they will happen. This is a left-brained idea. It is not wrong (or right for that matter), but it is limited. It is based upon the idea that our thoughts and intentions can directly affect an outcome. For example, if we hold in our minds the idea of something happening, say winning a million dollars, then the power of our intention will cause it to happen. This attributes a linear cause and effect process to something that is much more complex. The answer to all our problems does not lie in this type of magical thinking, just as it doesn't lie in logical scientific thinking or religious thinking ('I will pray to God who will sort this mess out').

Manifestation is much more complex and involves many steps. It involves us being open to our intuition and thereby receiving messages from our inner self about our direction. Once we understand that our inner self knows what is going on, we can use this information to plan our lives, or our path, or our way out of a problem. Firstly, we receive the information (yin fire that relies upon air, earth and water to receive). Then we use the power of our yang fire to act on it and create. We may be creating new ideas, or a physical work of art, or a new job, or a relationship, or a family. We may be creating any number of things, based upon the needs of our inner self. We create these things not just by thinking that they will happen but by organising our lives so they will happen.

Fire is the driving force and so when our inner self wants to manifest something it will drive us to do so in whatever way it can. If our inner self is not driving us then usually the project will not manifest. We may think we want to do something, or create something, but unless our inner fire is alight, we will not be successful. We will have enormous trouble manifesting it. Conversely, sometimes our inner fire drives us to do things that we think we don't want to do.

This is why fire has so much power. It can create wonderful things but it can also destroy things. Destruction usually happens because we are not aware of our inner needs, as if we are sabotaging ourselves in some way, working against ourselves. We sometimes destroy the very things we thought we wanted to create because our inner self has needs that it will always try to have met.

Some of these needs are to create but some are also to destroy the parts of our life that it considers no longer useful. The passion that drives a love affair is almost irresistible and it can destroy a marriage. The passion to create a work of art can take us to the brink if we forget that we also have other needs that aren't quite as irresistible.

Too much fire

People who have a lot of fire in their makeup sometimes have trouble living in the physical world. The most dramatic of these are people with bipolar disorder who have episodes of mania. These people have grand plans, big picture schemes; they are full of passion and creativity but it is ungrounded. They have lost touch with living in a physical world, are unable to carry out the grand plans, because they cannot break the plan down into small enough tasks to be able to take it on.

People in the grip of a manic episode are almost consumed by the yang fire. They appear larger than life and are very charismatic. They have brilliant ideas but generally, the ideas are very right brained. They are in touch with the holistic view of things and full of the spiritual fire energy but they are out of touch with the left brain and the limits of a physical world. They are unable to put the fire energy to use because they have lost touch with their earth side – logical thinking and planning, physical limitations.

Many of us slip into this space sometimes in our lives. It is common when we begin to be spiritually aware or become aware of our previously forgotten intuitive abilities. Then we may tend to go overboard and forget that our rational brain has its uses. So many 'spiritually aware' people swing too far into the light (fire and right-brained air). This is all part of the process of finding out who we are. We believed we were primarily physical and then we discover our spiritual side. It is a natural process that we explore this side of ourselves but we often forget what we have already learnt about the physical side of life.

We are filled with passion and bliss. Our fire burns brightly, but fire without air just burns itself out. We are always seeking greater balance and as we discover more about our fire, we need to balance it with our air side. The brain is designed to be used whole. In Western society, we learn how to use the left side. Then we discover that the right side is very useful too and we begin to perceive the world in different ways. We become more enlightened, we become more aware of our parts, of who we are. But if we overbalance into this new world view then we are forgetting what we have learnt about linear processes and logic. As we seek wholeness, we seek greater balance. Too much fire can be more destructive than too little.

Usually the problem with too much fire is that we have too much yang fire – too much drive to create. Sometimes, we have too much yin fire – we rely upon our intuition too much and forget that we also have physical senses that give us valuable information. Sometimes our intuition needs to be backed up by information that is more concrete. When I see a patient, I rely on my intuitive abilities and I look at them, listen to them and usually touch them (physically examine them) in order to get a fuller picture of their individual problems.

Too little yin fire

Most of us don't take advantage of our yin fire – our intuitive abilities. These abilities are throughout our body. We use the intuitive abilities of our right brain, our body and our feelings in order to process and understand the yin fire.

Accessing intuition is a natural process, however many of us have forgotten how to do it. It happens best when we manage to turn off our left brain and our logic, which usually tell us that intuition just doesn't make logical sense. It is not a linear process but a non-linear one. Intuition works because we are all connected via a giant web of ether. Physicists call this the quantum hologram; religions might call it the Holy Spirit. Whatever it is (I will discuss it more in the next chapter), it connects us invisibly. We receive information through this web or quantum hologram and it comes to us via our internal senses – our intuition. We can access this intuition through inner sight – dreams, daydreams, and visions; through inner hearing – thoughts, epiphanies, sudden understandings and insights; and through feelings – gut feelings, bodily sensations and emotional insights.

Some of us do this more naturally when we sleep. Our sleep hours are a time when our intuition is at work, so dreams are an intuitive process. The time between waking and sleeping is a good time to pay attention to your intuition. In the half-awake state when the left brain hasn't fully woken up, the right brain will often be communicating with your consciousness.

When we are awake, we need to more consciously access our intuition, or at least be open to it. We get intuitive flashes all the time but mostly we ignore them. Flashes, sudden insights and epiphanies are intuition. Then there are deliberate attempts to engage intuition through meditation or visualisation, and specific tools to engage intuition such as tarot cards or runes.

All of these are just techniques. Once we learn how to better access our intuition and use our intuitive thinking, we can learn how to use it more consciously in everyday life.

As we begin to tune in to our intuition, we find that the answers it gives us come suddenly and with a clarity that confounds our left-brain way of thinking. We suddenly understand a problem we have been grappling with, or the significance of last week's events suddenly dawn on us, or we realise we have been stuck in the same old pattern of dysfunctional behaviour with our partner and that it is up to us to change.

Intuitive thinking is like magic because we aren't conscious of the process, yet suddenly we find an answer. While sometimes it seems that the answer was staring us in the face all along, it isn't until we intuitively understand it that it makes sense to us.

Many times in the writing of this book, I grappled with a problem about some issue. My left brain was like a dog with a bone trying to get an answer. Then I'd just let it go, my intuition would kick in, and I would think, 'Oh I get it,' and understand the whole thing.

Both sides of the brain are working at the same time but we mainly pay attention to our left brain because it makes the most noise. The right brain tends to do its job quietly, whereas the left brain is always chattering away. We need to use both sides of the brain together but in order to learn how to do this better we need to disengage the left side so we can hear the right. This is where intuitive tools, meditation and the like come into play. They help us learn how to quieten the left side and pay attention to the right side and our other intuitive senses.

As we become better at paying attention to our intuition, we learn how to use it in all situations, how to combine our logical thinking and our intuitive thinking. This is how our brains were designed to be used – it is just that Western society has taught us how to be left-brain dominant (or we have taught Western society how to be left-brain dominant).

Too little yang fire

Most of us have lots of yang fire. In Western society, yang fire is encouraged – build more, create more, do more. This is at the expense of yin fire. We create from our thoughts what is right and wrong rather than from an inner knowing of what we need to create.

Sometimes we go through periods of too little yang fire. Typically, this is a period of depression. We end up earthbound, with no passion for life. Such periods may last for varying amounts of time. Sometimes they serve to bring us back to earth when we have become too filled with spirit. Our passion and creativity have not been adequately grounded in the earth, or we have been fulfilling someone else's dreams instead of our own, or we have spent too long on something that we are no longer as passionate about.

Too little fire leads to flatness in our lives, a lack of joy and enthusiasm for life. When we enter such a period we lose touch with the passion in our lives, and having lost touch with it, sometimes it's very hard to find it again.

Why do such periods of depression happen to so many of us? Why is there an epidemic of depression in our society? Is it because we have forgotten what really makes us happy, or that we lead our lives based upon expectations of society and a culture that doesn't put the whole person first? We lose touch with that part of ourselves that makes life joyful.

To regain our fire we need to make an effort to find what our passions are and begin to feed them. Sometimes it takes a long time to do this but it is often the best way out of depression.

Ways to pay better attention to your intuition

Our intuition is helpful for many things. In terms of fire, it is most helpful for generating ideas in order to direct our yang fire. It is also good for working out problems and controlling chaos in our lives, for finding new directions and for challenging beliefs.

Most of us have forgotten how to pay attention to our intuition, our inner self. We rely on what we perceive with our physical senses and our conscious awareness rather than also relying upon our inner knowing.

Essentially our conscious awareness looks outward. It focuses on things in the external world by using ego. Ego is that bridge between the conscious and the unconscious. Typically, in Western society we focus our attention on the external world. If we are to be whole people, we need to pay as much attention to our internal world and bring our inner knowing into our consciousness. We do this by accessing our intuition. We have to do this consciously at first until we get so good at it that we do it without even thinking.

The information from our inner self is available whenever we need it, but most of us do not believe this. We do not trust ourselves to know, so we need to begin by learning how to trust our inner self.

1. Dreams

Believing that our inner self sends us messages through dreams may take an enormous leap of faith. It means not only trusting in ourselves but also trusting in a part of ourselves that we would normally discount as being unreliable.

Dreams bring some of our unconscious knowledge to our conscious awareness. They do this in several ways. Sometimes it just happens as we spend time dreaming. At other times, it brings the dream to our conscious awareness and we are left wondering about the meaning. Sometimes we need to think about the meaning, other times it comes to us easily. Dream interpretation is useful for some people and not for others.

If you want to use your dreams as a way of finding answers to your problems, you need to begin believing that it is possible and then start looking at your dreams. As you interpret your dreams, it is best to do so symbolically rather than logically or literally. This symbolic interpretation is about looking at the meaning behind the dreams, examining the symbols and metaphors. When dreams really stick in our minds that is when it is most useful to have a deeper look at them. When dreams are recurring, our intuitive mind is attempting to get the message across even more strongly.

Sometimes, dreams send us clear messages that don't require much interpretation. Recently, I dreamt I was on a train travelling across Japan. We had some difficulty getting onto the train but once we were on it, we enjoyed a wonderful trip across the country. At every point, there was something to see or be involved in. We stopped at numerous places and each time we stopped the local people would be there doing something or offering us some entertainment. I said to my daughter, 'You see, it's the journey that's important not the destination.' I woke up with those words in my mind and the interesting thing was that this echoed events that had happened in the previous few days. Life is a journey.

2. Daydreaming

Daydreaming is an intuitive function that takes us out of our logical left brain. When we daydream we are absent in a sense, not part of what is going on around us. Off in our own little world, we seem to be disconnected from our conscious mind.

Sometimes this may be escaping from the realities of what is going on around us, as with children in school who aren't interested in what is happening or can't connect with the lesson. At other times, we are just taking time out.

Whatever the reason, when we daydream we often connect with our intuition and receive information that we might not usually be so good at receiving. In a way, it is similar to meditation but mostly it happens without any planning. We can plan time to daydream. We often daydream best when we are outside, especially in natural places. On holidays when we have time, we often dream about how our lives might be better but when we return to our everyday lives, we switch back to a rational mindset that gives us many reasons why our lives should stay as they are.

Pay attention to your daydreams in the same way as you pay attention to dreams when you are sleeping. Both are from your inner self.

3. Meditation

Meditation seems confusing because there are so many different ways that people do it. At its basis is the letting go of ego control and the seeking of our inner self. We open up our ego bridge to the inner self and allow it to talk to us. We quieten our conscious mind's judgements and beliefs about what is truth, allow ourselves to be open to our inner wisdom, listen to it and act upon it.

Meditation is just one way to be in better touch with our inner selves but it is not compulsory.

For those of us whose minds race along at a thousand thoughts a minute we will often have trouble quietening our brains. Classic meditation, where you sit or lie and go into a relaxed state and try and empty your mind, may be beyond us, or for some, not particularly useful. There is no doubt that the relaxed physical state has benefits for our body and that emptying the mind or being able to let the thoughts go has benefits for our health. But many people find classic meditation too different from their everyday life to bother with it.

An active meditation may suit them better because the rhythmic nature of exercise seems to shut off the brain eventually. Any exercise that is repetitive and rhythmic and that uses both sides of the body can be a meditative experience.

It is most important to be aware that there is no right way to meditate. Whatever you find best for you is the right way.

It may also help to focus on that time between wakefulness and sleep (both as you fall asleep and as you wake up). This altered state of consciousness is similar to deep meditation and if you practise trying to remain conscious in this state (rather than falling asleep), you may find your intuitive messages coming through.

I find that I get most of my answers in the time of semi-wakefulness, or when walking. My mind is not quiet in either state, but it is somewhat disengaged. It has stopped searching for the logical answer and it is more open to the inner self.

Remember that there is no one right way to do anything. What you are trying to do is to access your inner self, the wisdom and the intuitive knowing that it contains. Find your own way.

4. Intuitive tools

There are many intuitive tools available. Tarot, I Ching, angel cards, goddess cards, runes, a page from the Bible, crystal balls.

I have chosen to focus on tarot and runes because they are the ones I mostly use.

These tools have been designed to free our intuition from the restrictions of ego and the left brain so that we may see its messages more clearly. The greatest restriction (and the most common) that ego employs is to immediately label all these things as rubbish and not worth looking into. Left brainers will find it difficult to accept such things. If they open their minds enough to try, they will still often rationalise the whole experience and discount it.

All intuitive tools are just tools; they don't have magical powers. Intuitive tools help us learn how to access our intuition better. As we use them and learn more about the intuitive process, we can often let the tools go and access our intuitive thinking directly.

I don't use intuitive tools a lot of the time, but when I am stuck and focusing too much on my left-brain thinking, I reach for the tarot or the runes. When I see patients who are stuck, I encourage them to use an intuitive tool to help access their intuition.

Tarot

Tarot cards and packs have been around for hundreds of years. The pack is made up of 78 cards – 22 major arcana cards and 56 minor arcana cards. Arcanum means mystery or secret and lets us know that the use of these cards is a mystery and therefore not defined by logical rational explanations.

The 22 major arcana cards symbolise our journey through life and signify major life events or transitions. The minor cards are similar to a normal playing deck involving four suits of 14 cards, with ace through to king. Cards one (ace) to 10 are known as pip cards and the court cards are page, knight, queen, and king (thus giving us one more card in each suit than a normal playing deck). The minor cards deal more with our day-to-day existence and the way we react to our circumstances. A reading with many major cards will usually indicate a more important life transition than a reading with mostly minor cards.

The four suits are cups, wands, swords, and pentacles. Cups are linked with water, our feelings and emotions. Wands are linked with fire, our intuition and our passions. Swords are linked with air and the intellect. Pentacles are linked with earth and the body, the practical things in life.

All readings take into account our elements – fire, water, air, and earth – through the cards of the minor arcana. Ether is the connection between all the cards and is interpreted by looking at the linkages between the cards chosen. The major cards symbolise our soul's journey and the process we go through.

It is possible to use the tarot in many different ways. Most people will start by having a tarot reading where someone else (who knows the symbolism of the tarot) will interpret the meanings of the cards. While this is a good way to start, I think if you are going to use the tarot to tap into your intuition you are better off buying a good pack of tarot cards and a book that gives you the interpretations. Everyone uses their intuition to interpret the cards personally in a reading so the book is just a guide.

There are numerous types of tarot packs, all with different images on the cards. It is best to pick a pack that you like the look and feel of and then to become familiar with the images.

I use a variety of books but my favourite is Seventy-eight Degrees of Wisdom by Rachel Pollack.[14] It explains in some depth the symbolism behind each card and the journey through the major arcana cards. It might be a bit daunting for some beginners but it is a great reference.

Pick a tarot book that appeals to you; trust your intuition.

14   Details in Bibliography.

Runes

Runes are over 2,000 years old but many of their traditional meanings have been lost. The pack I use has 25 rune stones and a book of interpretations.[15] This is a fairly new interpretation of rune lore but it provides me with a way to reflect on the process of my life.

Using runes is simple – I just pull a rune out of the bag and read its message. Invariably, some parts of the message will attract me more than others and I pay more attention to these parts. It is also useful to leave the rune out for a while and re-read the interpretation. You can use runes for spreads in similar ways to tarot but I find tarot more useful in a spread because of the interconnectedness of the tarot cards.

There are many other intuitive tools around – use your intuition to pick one that appeals to you.

Ways to increase your yang fire

1. Pay attention to the physical

Yang fire needs to be grounded, so it is important to pay attention to the physical when you lack yang fire. The best ways to do this are to look after your physical body – exercise, eat well and get enough rest. As well as this, it's important to avoid artificial stimulants. While these seem to increase yang, artificial stimulation always leads to depletion of energy in the end. Another way to pay attention to the physical is to stay in tune with the cycles of the earth. Pay attention to night and day, to the seasons and to the weather.

2. Do more of what you love to do

Doing what you love is the best way to increase your yang fire. This is about exploring your passions, whether they seem creative outlets

15   'The Book of Runes', Ralph Blum. Details in Bibliography.

or not. Many of us spend our lives doing things for other people and forgetting about our own passions and creative outlets. Sometimes we need to discover what it is that makes our hearts sing and our passions stir. To do this we may need to use our intuition or we may just need to try new things.

At some level, we all know those things that we love to do even when we are in the midst of depression and despair. Sometimes we don't believe we deserve to do the things we love. We might feel that life is so dark that there is no light available to us. It is at these most difficult times that we most need to find our passions. We might need to start small and each day, do some small thing that brings us pleasure. Gradually, we build on this until we can recapture our passion for life. I know this is not an easy thing to do when we are down and feel flattened by life's circumstances, but increasing our yang fire is the best way out of depression.

At times, people feel that embracing their passions and doing what they love is selfish. In a way it is, but it is an important part of living whole. We can only bring our true gifts to the world when we are whole and developing our passions.

If you are having trouble connecting with your passions, then try writing them down. You may need to be very specific. At some point as you write down your ideas, you will notice a more positive emotional response to some ideas than to others. Follow these. The things that excite you and stir up your emotions are what bring you most joy. These are the passions we must follow.

3. Connect with others who share your passions

Sometimes we have trouble igniting our passions, especially if we have denied them for a long time or we are in the midst of depression. While it is good to connect with others at any time, it is especially important if you are having trouble. Depressed people are usually lacking yang fire and they have difficulty connecting with their passion and joy. If we can first identify some of our passions, we can then begin to connect with other people who share those passions. This is a good way to bring more joy to our life. It is a difficult thing to do in the midst of depression but as we begin to take more responsibility for our health, we see that we are the only person who can heal us.

Depression is endemic in our society and a large part of it is our disconnection with our inner self and with who we really are. We are trying to be someone else. In depression, we need to find ourselves in order to heal our pain. To do this we usually need to increase our fire, both our connection with our intuition and our connection with our passion. Depression is primarily about a lack of joy. If we can make a move to connect with others who are passionate, we begin the journey towards igniting our own passions.

Many people who are not depressed are still not connected with their yang fire and this is usually because they haven't given themselves permission to live their passion. But living our passions is what we are here to do. We find joy in this and we therefore bring joy and healing to others.

4. Access your intuition

I have written about this at length in the previous section, but accessing intuition is not just a yin activity. Yang fire often needs the yin for inspiration so you need to access your intuition in any way you can in order to find your own inspiration.

If you are at a loss to know what your real passions are then you need to ask your intuition for help. Simply acknowledging that you would like more joy and passion in your life will help you discover more about yourself. Give yourself permission to explore and discover, because this is our life-long journey. We do things we don't enjoy and we realise we want less of that in our life. We do things we do enjoy and acknowledge to ourselves that we would like more of those things. Our passions and the things that bring us joy change over time. Depression sometimes arises when we forget that we are changing beings and that what brought us joy and filled us with passion when we were 20 no longer does it for us when we are 50. This is called change and we always need to be open to changing our life around to fit in with what brings us more joy. When we follow where our passion leads, we begin to live the life we came here to live. But we have to believe that is so.

5. Stay centred

Staying centred means that we try not to go overboard when we follow our passions. Sometimes we will follow a single passion and we learn that it doesn't bring us as much joy as when we stay centred and pay attention to all our passions. We are not one-dimensional beings. We do not have one passion that we must follow at the cost of everything else; that is where some of us become unbalanced. When we become inspired by a creative urge, we sometimes forget we must also nourish other parts of our lives. Staying centred reminds us of this.

We follow our passions while remaining aware. We pay attention to our inner guidance and our intuition, which let us know if we are not centred or grounded. We pay attention to our physical symptoms. If we go overboard following a passion, we may forget that we need to sleep or eat, or that we need to nurture our relationships. Too much yang fire can be very destructive so we need to control this by remaining balanced and centred. This can be hard to do. When we first fall in love and are overcome with passion for the other person, we sometimes become so caught up in the situation that everything else in our world seems insignificant. This is how our passions capture our attention and make us follow them. At some point, the passion needs to be earthed or it will consume everything. As we follow our passions, we try to remain grounded and stay centred.

FIVE - ETHER

In the last few centuries, science has discovered much about our world and about how it works. It has done this using the scientific principle of reductionism. This concept takes a system and reduces the system to its constituent parts in the hope of discovering how the system works. This is a typical left-brain way of processing information.

We take a human body and reduce it to its various lesser systems: the cardiovascular system, the neurological system, the gastrointestinal system, and so on.

We then look at the components of one of these systems, for example, the cardiovascular system. This system is made up of the heart, the blood vessels, the blood, and so on.

Going down a layer further, we look at the tissues that make up these parts and the cells that make up these tissues.

Deeper down are the components of the cell – the cell wall, the cell contents such as the nucleus and mitochondria.

We break the system down into smaller and smaller parts hoping to discover how the system works and how we can fix it when it breaks.

When we get to the realm of quantum physics, which investigates the smallest particles that go to make up matter, we discover that the whole world is made up of only a few very small particles.

A human is made up of the same particles as a chair and a tree. Although we discover many things when we reduce a human to its smallest parts (or the smallest parts so far discovered), we do not discover much about the whole person. All we discover is that everything in the physical world is made up of the same sub-atomic particles.[16]

In many ways, reductionism is the opposite of holism. In holism, we consider the whole system. In reductionism, we consider the parts of the system. Yet the parts are just as important as the whole – the system relies on the parts and the parts rely on the system. Like yin and yang, the parts and the system are intertwined.

The mystery of life lies in the whole person, the whole plant, the whole earth, the whole universe. Who we are is determined by our parts and by the way the parts are combined. How the parts are combined and how all the parts of the system we call earth are combined is via something called ether. This is part of the mystery of life and humans have been trying to define it for centuries. What is ether? What is this unifying force that connects us all and flows through us?

I have chosen to call this element ether but we might just as well call it spirit. Spirit for me, however, has religious overtones. For most of my childhood, I went to church every Sunday and I took on many of the beliefs that my church held. In my teenage years, I became a fervent Christian but it quickly became apparent that this belief system was not for me.

Many people brought up in a religious culture have trouble with the idea of God and Spirit because those words have a certain meaning. Spirit in my religious upbringing was the Holy Spirit and

---

16   This is an oversimplification. I explore more about the theoretical underpinnings of holism in Part three.

was one of the three parts of God – Father, Son and Holy Spirit. God, the father, was like a man sitting up in heaven watching over us, a somewhat punitive figure who decided whether you went to heaven or hell based upon your goodness or lack of it. The Holy Spirit was that part of God that moved within people and helped them be god-like.

I choose to call the fifth element ether because it has no religious overtones.

Ether is mysterious yet physicists have discovered its presence and they call it 'zero point energy' and the 'quantum hologram'.

Zero point energy is the energy that molecules retain even at absolute zero of temperature (minus 273.17 degrees Celsius or zero on the Kelvin scale). Even when molecules should be frozen in space, they are still moving. Of course, quantum mechanics has as one of its 'rules' that no object (in sub-atomic terms) can ever have precise values of location and velocity at the same time.[17] This is a classic paradox and holism is full of them.

Ether, then, is the presence of energy even at the point in a physical universe when you would expect there to be no energy.

The idea of the quantum hologram came together from the work of various physicists. It suggests that a unifying force (zero point energy) joins the universe holistically. The process of interconnectedness is one of non-local resonance through the zero point field. This non-local connectedness means that at the quantum level there can be transfer of information (which might include thoughts, feelings and intentions) throughout the universe instantaneously.

The whole idea of the universe being linked through this quantum hologram is a bit mind blowing but it fits with Eastern theories of

17   See Part three for more on the physics.

Qi and prana, with traditional American Indian ideas of a web of life and with Australian Aboriginal ideas of dreamtime. This is not a new idea; it is just that physicists have 'discovered' its presence on the sub-atomic level.

Ether is the element that connects us all in this invisible web. It connects our parts, it connects us to other people and things, and it connects us in ways that we don't understand.

We can easily feel how we are connected to people and things on a physical level as we interact with them, but ether works on a deeper level and we are largely unaware of it. Imagine that there is a giant web on a microscopic level and that its filaments connect us to everyone else and everything else on earth. It goes beyond this, but let's imagine it at a level that we can make sense of. These filaments carry information between us all and the information travels instantaneously.

All day we are receiving information through this web of filaments, and we are sending it out. This giant web connects us all. Everything we do, think, and feel is transmitted into the web. Everything that others do, think and feel can be transmitted to us.

We are not alone.

We are not the separate beings that we Westerners believe.

The Chinese use the name *Qi* (pronounced Chi) to encompass their ideas about ether. Indians use the word *prana* and the system of chakras. Homeopaths conceptualise it in terms of *miasms*. Each of these is a way to conceptualise something that is beyond our logical understanding. This is critical to a real understanding of the concept of ether – we can't understand it logically, we can only understand it on an intuitive level. Until our right brain can grasp the whole of it, we won't understand it. I can explain it as much as I like in logical terms but because it isn't a logical phenomenon, this does not lead to a proper understanding.

Ether encompasses the connections between all things: between our different parts, between us and our neighbour, between us and our enemy, between us and the earth.

Everything we do has the potential to affect the web. We can alter the quantum hologram by altering our self. Yet the paradox is that everything everyone else does can alter the web, the quantum hologram, and this can affect us on a personal level.

So where does that leave us? Are we totally at the mercy of the quantum hologram? Is this the physicist's idea of God? Who is in charge? Who is running the show?

In holistic terms, there is no one thing or person running the show. We are all running the show – together. This is a mighty scary thought because we aren't very good at looking after one planet, much less a universe and beyond. However, in holistic terms we only have to do our part. We don't have to run the whole show. We don't have to fix everything, we just have to play our part in the web.

To play our part we have at our fingertips the giant resource of the quantum hologram. Through the ether we can find everything we need to know, but we have to learn how.

Ether works whether we are aware of it or not. We are intricately enmeshed in the web of life, we are part of the quantum hologram, we are not separate from everything else. When we pretend that we are, the system fragments. We believe in our conscious minds that we are separate, so the information that we receive via the ether tends to support this belief. We cut ourselves off from the resources of our inner self, which is connected to the quantum hologram, but the inner self and the quantum hologram are always agitating to break into our consciousness. The process of life is always trying to get our attention.

SIX -
THE PROCESS OF LIFE

So far, I have tried to separate content and process in order to describe them. This is an attempt to understand something using mechanistic reductionist principles and it never gives us the whole picture. All we get is some understanding of the bits, yet no real understanding of the whole thing.

The bits are the content. The cycles that life undergoes are the processes. Together they make a whole, but understanding the whole does not just mean understanding the bits and the process. We can never grasp the whole through logical thinking and models; we can only understand the whole by experiencing it. Likewise, when we experience it we can never capture the experience. Language and symbols are only ever representations of the whole because an integral part of the whole is the process. Process is movement and change. Nothing ever stays the same; everything is impermanent on some level.

In order to heal ourselves we need therefore to not only find our own balance – our unique self – but also be aware that this self is not stable. Our self is always changing. We attempt to discover who we are, but who we are is not one set thing, we are changing, transforming, growing. We are part of a much larger system that is also changing and transforming.

Western medicine has assumed that the content of the human system and the processes that occur within the system can be separated. Holistic medicine assumes that content and process are connected.

While this chapter is about the processes within and around systems, keep in mind that we can't really separate the process completely from the content of the system. They are connected in ways we don't yet understand.

I would first like to discuss the two main processes that are going on all the time.

The first is linear. This is the one we are most comfortable with. Cause and effect.

The second is non-linear, the process of chaos. We don't particularly like this one because we don't know how to control it.

Both processes are occurring at the same time and are interwoven and connected. Linear processes typically occur along a time line and are relatively easy to control if we are fully aware of the inputs required. If we want to become a doctor then the linear process that occurs is that we have to get really good marks at school, then get into medical school and then get through five or six years of medical training. The process occurs over time and has various essential elements.

Much of contemporary life has developed along these lines. This is because Western society (and those of us who live in it) loves linear process. We would love it if life were only linear (in fact our culture often pretends that life is only linear), however linear processes are often interrupted by chaos. This can be a mini chaos that doesn't interfere with the linear process but rather accompanies it. An example would be where the medical student is going along fine in their medical course, on their way to becoming a doctor, but their personal life is in tatters. Their boyfriend has left them and they are emotionally distraught.

Generally in this situation the student is able to continue with the linear process (the medical course) while battling against the chaos around them. From a holistic point of view, the linear process and the chaos are in some ways connected but we usually prefer not to make any connection between them.

Sometimes chaos will intervene in a more dramatic manner. The boyfriend leaves because of the demands of the medical course. This may then directly affect the linear process, which now also enters chaos. The medical student is forced to face the connectivity of it all and the interrelatedness of all parts of their life.

Many of us are quite proficient at solving linear problems. We use our logical analytical problem-solving skills and find answers. Few of us are proficient at solving non-linear problems. Most of the 'problems' that we feel so 'stuck' in are usually chaotic in nature.

The process of chaos is nature's way (soul's way, evolution's way) of pushing us towards our full potential, our wholeness. Chaos is designed for growth and expansion. It seeks to teach us how best to combine all our aspects to become whole, to become who we really are. The story of our life reflects the process of aligning our physical self with our spiritual self in order to become whole.

Our physical self rules our conscious awareness. As we grow and evolve, our spiritual (or inner) self gradually becomes accessible to our conscious awareness and so we grow as we access more of our inner knowledge. The physical, external self and the spiritual, internal self are not actually separate, but as we become aware of their existence, we see them initially as two separate parts.

Chaos, life, growth, everything, is a process that has no beginning and no end. There is no outcome, no end to the process, no happy ever after. There is only more process that leads to more growth and more expansion of awareness.

If this sounds exhausting and you already feel that you need a rest, that's fine. You do need a rest because that's part of the process. The same as we have awake and asleep times, a deciduous plant has a dormant phase in winter. The cycle of any process relies on periods where growth is hidden or dormant. The cycle of life is birth, growth, death, decay, fertilisation, gestation, birth and then more growth. In fact, the cycle of life is more like a spiral as we grow and evolve. We return to a place we have already been but we have learnt a little more, evolved a little more, so that we never really return to exactly the same place.

The process of our lives is not difficult unless we try to make it so. It is a completely natural process and it has its own rhythms. As we learn how to allow ourselves to undergo the process, we learn how easy it can be. All we have to do is live our lives.

More often than not, we want to reach an outcome. We want the process over. We want the answer. And we want it all right now.

We try to force it, we try to speed up the process and alter it in innumerable ways so that we have more control.

Let's look at how we make our lives harder than they need to be by trying to alter the natural process of chaos.

One way we do this is by reverting to limiting beliefs (logical, linear thinking).

The three big limiting belief systems are that our reality is dictated either by God, by the intellect or by magic. These all limit us because they place our point of power within a limited range – within our left brain and its ideas of God, the intellect or magic.

We realise the process of chaos is occurring when things get uncomfortable. Something doesn't feel right, things aren't happening the way we planned, our life seems confused and is in upheaval.

Enter God (or rather our idea of God). We pray and pray, hoping for a particular outcome to this process that we find so uncomfortable. We forget to pay attention to our intellect, our body, our intuition and our feelings but rely for an outcome on the idea that something outside of us will rescue us from our predicament.

Alternatively, enter intellect that thinks it can logically sort out this mess we are in by pure reasoning, by rationally taking the problem to pieces and solving it, or by getting someone else (an expert) to do it for us (doctors, counsellors, friends, family).

Alternatively, enter our magical thinking. We believe that by dint of positive imagery and the power of our intention we can sort out this mess. If only I could believe it, I could heal myself.

Sometimes we try all three ways at once.

My personal favourites might play out as follows.

I am in love with a man who seems to want to end our relationship.

I might appeal to God in the form of angels to intercede on my behalf to get this man to change his mind.

Alternatively, I sit and think about what I could do to make a difference. I go over many scenarios in my mind trying to work out what is logically going on. I believe that if only I could work out where we went wrong then he would want to keep trying.

I might use my magical thinking to visualise a new start to our relationship. I try to believe that this is possible and that the only reason it doesn't happen is because I don't believe it strongly enough, or I am not good enough at visualising the outcome I want.

Then I try a little prayer to the angel of relationships to help prod him along.

I try to talk to him and have a rational discussion about why we should keep seeing each other.

Finally, I ask my intuition for help and I do a rune reading. This tells me I should stop trying to control the process so much.

I stop for a while and just live the process, going with the flow, doing what feels right. However, nothing happens so I start praying to the angels again and rationalising again and doing more creative visualisation.

I am making it all harder on myself than it needs to be because I am unable to trust the process of my own life. I am unable to trust that I (my inner self) know what is happening, that I am going in the direction I need to go, that what I am going through is how I will learn what I need to learn.

The conscious I, my smaller self, has no idea what I need to learn. My inner self (soul) has an idea of what I need to learn but even it may not know it exactly. It just knows with the help of its spirit aspect how to put me in the right situation so I am most likely to learn it efficiently.

Sometimes I fear that either my inner self is wrong or that I am an exceedingly slow learner, for it seems to me that it takes me years to learn one thing. Maybe that is just how it is or maybe I am not always aware of how much I learn when I let the process happen without trying to control it. Maybe my attempts at controlling the process in some way hinder my learning.

Certainly, part of what I am learning is how to trust the process better. I am learning how to allow my elements to mix themselves in soul's way and not automatically jump in with more ether or more intellect or more intuition. I am learning more how not to block my own process through fixating so hard on a desired outcome.

Relinquishing control

A patient with depression recently came to see me. A psychiatrist had diagnosed her with severe depression and put her on antidepressants. She felt out of control. She couldn't stop thinking, couldn't function in her normal life.

Western society and medicine treat depression with drugs to inhibit the process and provide 'talking' therapy to try to help the patient gain control of their mind. This is an attempt to control things on the physical level but what it actually does is attempt to control the patient's process. Medicine hates not to be in control.

What if the problem is due to fragmentation and lack of wholeness? What if the problem is that this woman's inner self is so completely swamped by the physical world that the only way it can get attention is to erupt (increasing the energy)?

The outcome the inner self wants is quite different from the outcome the ego wants. The ego wants control back. It wants the old safe way of life; it cannot understand what went wrong. The soul wants to be heard; it wants this woman to undergo the process to discover more about her whole self.

This woman, like us all, has at least two choices. The first is the path of science and logic. This is the familiar, relatively safe path she has trodden for the past 35 years. She could just as easily take the linear path of God or of magical thinking.

She takes the logical path of antidepressants and a therapist who tells her how she might think better. She gradually recovers and regains her old life. The depression has gone and she will have changed in some way, but has she learnt what her soul wanted? We have treated the physical aspect but ignored the spiritual; we haven't approached this in a whole person manner.

The second choice is to take the path of the soul. This is unfamiliar and possibly unsafe because it automatically challenges everything this woman's life has been based on up until now. The outcome in physical terms is completely unknown but in a spiritual sense is completely unimportant. The only outcome that matters to our soul is that we learn how to be truer to our essential nature and rediscover our wholeness.

The holistic path for this woman does not focus purely on physical outcomes. This is a giant step for most of us. How can we have faith in a process that might lead us anywhere at all?

Can this woman with depression take a different view?

Fortunately, she already had. She told me she understood that everything that was going on would lead her to a better place. She couldn't see how she was going to get there and it was frightening.

She thought she had to work it all out in her head (intellect) and when that led to even more confusion she thought a doctor might help. Doctors can help in many processes that we go through but the only way to have any control is to give up on the idea that we can rationally control such a process.

Our inner selves (souls) know what they are doing. The challenge is to pay attention to the process and not to panic.

My patient needed to stop her obsessive linear thinking because that type of thinking is not useful in this situation. She needed to realise that her left brain could not solve this particular problem.

She needed to pay more attention to her feelings and let them deliver their messages.

She needed to have some trust in her intuitive thinking, which would help her understand what her soul was asking for (an intuitive understanding, not a logical understanding).

She needed to make use of the etheric connections between her and everyone around her.

She needed to tap into the energy of spirit in any way she could.

What can I do as her doctor? I have to trust that my soul knows what is happening because I sure as hell can't work it out in my head. I have to avoid both our attempts to focus on a physical outcome. I have to resist my ego desire to control the process in some way. I have to pay attention to her process and my own process and not panic.

In a physical world, we think of outcomes as good or bad, right or wrong. In a physical world, we are always trying to solve a problem by controlling it. We are always taking a linear approach and heading for a desired outcome by trying to control what we think are the critical factors. What if we were to replace our linear approach with a chaotic approach?

How does a system of chaos reach an endpoint? It reaches it only when it has finished its process, when it gets to an outcome, and then it starts all over again.

The process of chaos goes on within us and around us, it is the process of life and we see it happening everywhere. It is the process whereby what we think of as chaos and destruction is also healing. What is being destroyed is our fragmentation and the fragmentation of things around us. This destruction via the process makes way for wholeness.

As a larger example, in Australia in 2007 we were in the grips of a severe drought.[18] Water, which many of us took for granted, became rare and precious. Our society was plunged into chaos as we tried to work out logically how we could avert further chaos (drought). Could we build bigger dams or pipes, could we use less water?

We use less water and look to government for answers to a problem that is much deeper than that. We pray for rain, we visualise rain, we use all of our combined logic to try to find an answer that will take us back to our old way of life, which is not to worry about water.

Taken as a chaotic process we might instead give ourselves up to the process, look to our intuitive powers to bring to our awareness how we have become fragmented and how we might heal that. In this sense, it is how we have become disconnected with nature. We have been fooled by our belief in a certain nature of reality, our belief that we are all separate and that what we do does not affect everything else.

---

18   We were when I wrote this chapter. In 2011, we had unprecedented floods.

The outcome we seek is to have as much water as we previously had. The outcome that the organism earth (of which we are all a part) is possibly working towards is healing, a step towards wholeness and away from fragmentation. In this way, the chaotic process of drought naturally brings people together in communities. It reminds us all that we rely on water, that we are connected, that the food we buy comes from farms that need water, that we are part of a greater whole that is the planet earth.

In this way, the process brings about healing. If however we focus solely on the outcome of more water and we build more dams and pipes, we miss the learning and the healing that is possible. We miss the bringing together of our parts to make us whole, the bringing together of the parts of this earth to make it whole again, the recognition that because we are all connected what we do affects everything else.

This is the process of chaos and the process of life. This process has at its basis an outcome of healing, of becoming whole or more balanced. Becoming whole is not just an endpoint so much as a beginning of a new cycle of growth and wholeness.

It's a bit like when we plant a seed. The seed grows and becomes a plant that flowers and sets seed and dies. We are left with the seed again, which has all the potential of its parent plant and more possibilities as well. It germinates and grows and the cycle repeats. The consciousness of the seed is dormant within the seed and it becomes manifest as it grows into its full potential – its wholeness if you like. In a sense, it was whole as a seed, or at least it was potentially whole, just as we are all potentially whole waiting to become fully whole. As we become whole, we fulfil our purpose, just as the plant did, our purpose being to become whole and the process of life being the process by which we achieve this wholeness (and then the cycle or spiral repeats itself).

In linear terms, we cannot grasp the enormity of this because it is not a linear process. As we allow ourselves to reach the potential of our wholeness, we begin to understand on an intuitive level what is going on. We raise our consciousness. Our potential expands. Our consciousness expands further.

The process of growth, the process of life, is chaos. How do we control it?

We don't. We allow it to have its way. This is how processes work; they have to occur. We search within the process for the meaning (which is an individual unique meaning). How am I not balanced; in what ways am I fragmented? We seek to bring to our awareness the ways in which we can heal ourselves.

With my patients, I try to help them see that there might be a different way of resolving their problems. To become whole rather than just a collection of parts we must own all of ourselves and remember that everything is interrelated. Our feelings affect everything else, just as our thoughts can. Problems with our physical body can affect our feelings and our thoughts; we can never fully separate each piece of ourselves and work on that area without taking into account how we are affected as a whole person.

How does each of us enter into the process better? How can we take advantage of the process?

Learning how to live the process of life often begins with logical attempts to understand it but until we begin to understand the process intuitively, we just don't get it. We may know in our left brain that everything is connected and that our feelings and intuition matter but until we know it in our whole self, it's all just theory. Before we go on to look at how we can practically live more holistically, let's look a bit more deeply at the theory.

PART THREE

HOLISTIC THEORY

It is not possible to solve an intractable problem using the same thinking that caused the problem in the first place.

Albert Einstein

ONE - THE CULTURE OF HOLISM

I began to think about writing this book many years ago. I had no idea what it was about; I just knew I had to write it. It was like a small fire inside me that grew with the passing years. However, my belief system told me I couldn't do it and for a long while I believed it. I was living and working in a culture that had its traditions and rules and for many reasons I found myself struggling.

As the circumstances of my life changed in my early forties, I found myself separated from my husband and without a job. I then started to write, most of it fiction, but sometimes I dabbled with the idea of a non-fiction book on healing. When I wrote I felt a strange peacefulness, but I still ignored the feeling that I needed to write about healing.

As I wasn't working, the money started to run out and I had to go back to work. It turned out the job I got was just the job I needed to help me build a framework for my ideas about healing. I worked as a sub-dean in a rural medical school with Melbourne University. Our job was to help train medical students to become doctors.

I learnt much more about the culture of medicine and about the beliefs behind this culture. I learnt a whole lot of things that I needed to learn in order to be able to write this book. My inner self was leading me (or to put it another way, the unconscious part of myself was leading the conscious part) but mostly I was following at a distance, kicking and screaming half the time because I thought I wanted to go somewhere else. I did want to go somewhere else, I just didn't realise I was going there anyway. If I had accepted the process and paid more attention, I might have got there a lot quicker (or not, I'm still not quite sure).

After about a year and a half as sub-dean, I realised that much of what we were teaching the students conflicted with what I believed in. The medical course focuses on the physical dimensions – the physical body and the intellect. I was coming to a greater understanding of the realms beyond the physical. Teaching from a reductionist physical viewpoint felt hypocritical.

While parts of the curriculum espoused treating the patient as a whole person, the course as a whole (and most of the people who taught it) operated from a biomedical, mechanistic perspective. For a while I stayed in the job thinking it was what I should be doing, thinking that they needed me, that I was doing a great job, so why not keep doing it? I managed to ignore the feelings of frustration that continually welled up inside me. I managed to discount the dreams of something different.

My soul was sending me messages to move on.

It was sending them in the form of thoughts – I don't want to do this anymore. Funny how we can talk ourselves out of that one.

It was sending them in the form of feelings – frustration, anger, grumpiness.

It was sending them in the form of my intuition – dreams and intuitive feelings that I could be doing something more personally meaningful than what I was doing.

My soul was sending me physical symptoms – more colds, aches and pains and tiredness.

And my soul was sending me messages via the ether – I was getting signs that I should change jobs.

But did I listen?

Not very well. I knew I wouldn't be staying in the job forever but I couldn't take the step of resigning. My ego was afraid of the change but liking the position of power that I found myself in. Sub-dean was a relatively powerful job so part of me was really enjoying that.

It was just after Angela died that I could no longer ignore the process of my life. This sudden and unexpected tragedy brought a new clarity to my life.

Part of the strength of our friendship had been our unconditional acceptance of each other. This was a bit unusual for both of us as we were fairly opinionated, judgemental and stubborn but in each other, we found a kindred spirit. She taught me such a lot about love yet we never talked about it. We just loved each other without ever having to analyse it or measure it. That was one of her gifts to me.

When she died, I felt extreme sadness but I knew her spirit was still around. The spiritual connections exist between us even when someone dies. These invisible connections manifest themselves as dreams, electrical malfunctions and strange co-incidences and despite all the sadness, a presence of love. Angela's death helped me realise that although our physical body dies, the love and spiritual connection does not.

At the time of her death, I went through a profound transformation. These transformations are difficult to describe in a rational logical way because they are experiential, not logical. We experience a sudden epiphany or understanding of some concept we have been struggling with. One of the things that I suddenly understood was that any of us could die at any time. I had known this intellectually before but I had never understood the significance in a personal sense, I had not integrated that intellectual knowledge into my being. I now understood that doing a job I didn't want to do was a waste of time. My soul had been trying to tell me this for a while but it took Angela's death for me to really understand the messages.

I realised that I had to quit my job and start writing again. It was then that I began to write this book.

The process of my life over the next year allowed me to clarify the movement from one world view to a different world view. I rewrote this book a number of times. At one stage, I had written about 80,000 words and thought the book was nearly finished. But my soul in its various ways told me that this was not so. Instead of rationalising that I had all these words written and surely they were useful, I listened to my inner self.

In a way I had to because my computer was doing all sorts of crazy things. I tried to work on the book but the screen would keep scrolling up and down and sections would highlight themselves. I changed the batteries in the mouse to no effect. I changed the mouse but still it kept happening. So I experimented. I began to delete the highlighted sections bit by bit. It made me dizzy because the words were still scrolling up and down but I just kept deleting.

In the end, I deleted 80,000 words and I was left with about 5,000. I still had the backup copies so it wasn't risky, but once I had done it the computer settled down. It stopped scrolling up and down and making me dizzy, so I figured that I was on the right track. I began to rewrite the book from a relatively blank slate.

I know this all sounds weird, but this sort of thing is what happens when we start to pay attention to the world spiritually (metaphysically). Previously I would have got very cross with the computer and become frustrated. Now I try to look beyond the physical to discover a deeper meaning. I don't yet understand this in a logical sense, probably because it has no rational explanation, or maybe we just haven't worked out the logic of these processes yet.

Once I had deleted all those words, I suddenly got new ideas about how to structure the book and what to write. I reused some of what I had previously written but it wasn't until I let go of it all that other ideas came into my mind.

The shift that is occurring within me is a shift from one culture to another. I am shifting from the culture of the physical to the culture of holism. It is a shift of world views.

This shift has allowed me to understand that I am not just a physical being. This is an intuitive understanding and therefore not logical. Such a thing cannot be scientifically proven in the context of our current scientific (logical) thinking. We continually grapple with such beliefs because they aren't logical, but on the intuitive level we know that we are partly spiritual and partly physical.

Because I am not just a physical being, because there is something beyond the physical, I have to learn the ways of this new culture. I also have to empty myself of many of the ways of the old culture in order to make way for the new.

This is what is termed a paradigm shift. I am moving from one paradigm or world view to another, and I am not alone. Many people are experiencing this shift and our society is on the edge of a major change. It is like moving from the trees to the ground, from an idea of the world as flat to the world as round. Now we are moving from the idea of the world as purely physical to the idea that the world is more than just physical.

These paradigm shifts are really shifts in consciousness. On an individual level, they indicate a growth in consciousness and when enough individuals grow in consciousness the paradigm shift occurs, the culture shifts and our basic belief system changes. As we undergo this cultural shift there may be many symptoms of cultural shock. We may feel all at sea, confused about the meaning of life, unsure where we fit into the world.

Our reality is constructed from our belief system, not because we construct what we believe but because we can only perceive what we believe. In a multi-dimensional reality, if we believe there are only three dimensions we can only perceive the three dimensions. Our soul is part of a multi-dimensional reality so it is always sending us evidence of other dimensions. At times we perceive some of these other dimensions, in our dreams, meditation, daydreaming, visions, creative inspirations, psychic messages. But mostly we are so convinced that the three-dimensional physical reality is the only true reality that we do not perceive the evidence of other realities.

The old culture, the one I am leaving, is based on the belief that reality is three-dimensional and therefore only physical. It believes that a person's identity is related to their physical body and their personality (our sense of personal identity, our ego consciousness). It believes that the intellectual mind, the concrete thinking left brain, is the keeper of truth. It believes that our physical bodies and the physical world are the only reality. It operates under a system of beliefs that many of us never question because we are not even conscious of it. We mistakenly consider our belief system to be reality or truth so we never think to question its validity.

This physical-based culture discounts the spiritual elements of us all. It denigrates feelings. It ignores intuition and it pays little attention to the connections between us and the energetic power of spirit. It believes in the idea of duality; that there is right and wrong and that fear and love are opposing forces. It believes that life is a linear process.

All of us live in this culture. Is it any wonder that most of us feel somewhat alienated, disconnected, separate, and fragmented? This is not who we really are. We are not really like this culture we have created.

This culture arose between 1500 and 1700. Before this, the prevailing world view of the Middle Ages might be called 'organic'. In the Middle Ages, society was made up of small communities that were tied to the land and therefore had a close relationship with nature. The people in such communities were dependent upon one another and on the land for their survival. Their religious and scientific beliefs were tied up with their beliefs about the natural world and their place in it. They lived the process of their lives more in tune with that natural world.

In the seventeenth century, the scientific revolution led to a paradigm shift in culture and belief systems. This new belief system came about through the scientific advances of Copernicus, Galileo and Newton and the ideas of Descartes. This scientific revolution led to the belief that the material universe and all its parts were like a machine. To investigate the universe as well as biological systems required reducing the systems to their relevant parts (reductionism). This mechanistic world view has continued to the present day. Although physics has developed theories and research indicating a new, more holistic or ecological world view, society and the biological sciences are still mainly operating from the mechanistic world view.

The mechanistic world view supports the belief that we are like machines and that we can control life through linear processes. Our society and culture are in transition. We are undergoing a paradigm shift from a mechanistic world view to a holistic world view. This shift occurs as the planet earth and its inhabitants undergo a major transition. It occurs partly through the process of chaos. It is no wonder that the earth seems to be in crisis, that our old ways of thinking and being no longer seem to work. This change is happening around us whether we like it or not; earth as a system is trying to heal herself.

The holistic culture is a new way of thinking and being and we are discovering it as we go. It cannot be described in logical neat terms and two-dimensional models like the old mechanistic culture. It will require new ways of thinking and new language to try to encapsulate it. It will have as its basis the idea that we are all connected – people, animals, earth, air – that everything is a system within a larger system and that all are interdependent. It will acknowledge the usefulness of both ways of thinking – intellect and intuition. It will pay attention to feelings and the physical. It will nurture the spiritual within us all and between us all.

Moving to a new culture means giving up our old ideas and starting to believe new ones. We do not know (our ego does not know, our brain does not know) what is best for us because we have been thinking we live in a purely physical world. We are not consciously aware of our path or of how our lives will unfold because if we were, there would be no point in the journey. Part of the meaning of the journey is that where we are going is not predetermined; the journey is the process by which we change and heal.

Where we are going is determined by the interplay between the inner and outer aspects of ourselves. Where we are going is not an endpoint or destination so much as a direction. We can base our direction on the physical aspects (externally) and we will follow one journey, or on both our internal and external aspects and we will find the path we are meant to travel.

The physical world is real, our bodies are real, and our minds are real. These things are not an illusion as some metaphysicians would have us believe. What is an illusion is that this is all we are. It is an illusion when we think and believe that we are just our bodies and just our minds. We all know, deep inside, that we are much more than this. We know it when we fall in love, when we create something beautiful, when we see beauty in others, when we give birth, when someone we love dies, or when we experience joy.

The mystical experience

While the presence of our soul (our spiritual nature) cannot be proven scientifically (partly due to our limited beliefs about scientific proof), this part of us has always been a prominent part of our lives. It is only in recent times that the soul has fallen into disrepute. Before the age of reason (scientific age), even Western society believed in the presence of the soul. Eastern traditions and native cultures have always been aware of our dual nature – physical and spiritual.

The mystical experience has always been considered evidence of this part of humans. While science would explain such experiences away by logical argument, the occurrence of any mystical experience is usually enough to convince the individual of the presence of spirit and soul.

A mystical experience is an experience where we are in touch with this spiritual part of ourselves and therefore in touch with spirit and the oneness of everything.

Mystics down through the ages have all described similar experiences. There is a radiance or brilliant light, a feeling of absolute peace and love, and an understanding that everything is connected and that in some sense everything is one.

Mystical experiences are by nature experiences and as such, they cannot be adequately described, but most of us at some stage in our lives have glimpsed this spiritual dimension. When we glimpse it, we gain an intuitive understanding of the oneness and immenseness of our spirit. This is an experience of holism.

What we all seek is to experience this holistic sense of ourselves most of the time. We seek to live as whole people, expressing both our spiritual and our physical individuality and at the same time consciously being part of a larger system.

Language of Holism

1. Metaphor

As with any new culture, we have to learn the language, the means of communication. When I began at medical school, I thought I would never understand the new foreign language that my teachers were talking. They spoke words that I had never heard before, but gradually the more I listened, the more I understood.

So it is with holism and metaphysics. This culture has its own language and its own form of communication. We don't really need to learn it so much as recognise it.

Physical language depends upon literal translation. Metaphysical or spiritual language depends upon figurative or metaphorical translation. In a way, this is like lateral thinking. We look at something not directly but sideways and see if we can get a different understanding of it. We try to see things differently.

We take a thought that has been going round and round in our head and see if it might have another meaning.

We read a story and understand that it has some meaning for us apart from its literal meaning.

We make a Freudian slip and take time to try to understand what it might mean for us personally.

We notice a song on the radio that seeks out our attention and we pay attention to the words and see if they tell us something.

We begin to notice that everything around us, as well as having a literal physical meaning, might also have a metaphoric, metaphysical meaning. We pay attention to the meaning and see where it takes us. Rather than identifying with words, our deeper self identifies with symbols and metaphors. Deeper still is pure thought and pure feeling but we are still learning about these things. First we must learn how to translate the symbolism into what we already understand.

The language of holism is exciting, like any new language, but it takes us a long time to become fluent. We keep reverting to our native tongue, the language of the literal, and we have to remind ourselves to do the translation. Gradually, as we translate everything, we begin to see things differently.

It has always intrigued me how someone who can speak more than one language thinks. Which language do they think in? When a French person is speaking English, are they translating it into French in their mind? At some stage the thinking must become English, and then a person really becomes fluent.

It is the same here. Learning the language of holism takes time and practice. The more you practise the more you begin to incorporate the language into your thinking. The way you think actually changes. Rather than relying totally on your concrete analytical brain, you begin to rely more on your intuitive brain. Gradually, you begin to see the meaning beneath the literal meaning in everything and you begin to enter other dimensions. The process happens at many levels – as we learn the language we enter the culture more and as we enter the culture more we learn the language.

Five years ago when my computer malfunctioned, I dismissed it as a stupid machine. When it acts up now, I pay attention and follow where it leads. The process of writing this book has been about trying to understand this new language and the new process. When something happens that I would have previously thought was inconvenient or frustrating, I try to look at it from a different viewpoint.

If my car breaks down when I am on my way to an important meeting, instead of becoming angry and trying to work my way out of my predicament I just try to sit with it. What part of me doesn't want to be at the meeting? Is there something about this meeting that doesn't get me started? Is my battery flat or have I run out of fuel? I let the anger flow through me until I understand it.

When I am frustrated with my partner and feel particularly stubborn about an issue, the symbolism of events sometimes gives me more information. I believe I am in the right and I'm not prepared to back down. Then the bull next door breaks through the fence and sits in my paddock eating the grass. He won't move, just stands there eating and no amount of shouting or pushing will budge him. When I see the symbolism, I begin to laugh because my soul and the universe have such a good sense of humour.

This new language becomes an interesting way to communicate with myself and with the universe. If I have a problem I look for the signs, symbols and metaphors that help me sort it out.

2. Paradox

Holistic language also embraces the idea of paradox. A paradox can be defined as something that seems to be contradictory and yet is possibly true.

A paradox cannot be understood by our left brain because paradox is not logical. Paradox is however central to the way the right brain thinks and the way soul works. Paradox is part of the new paradigm in the same way that the dualistic idea of right and wrong is part of the old one.

The paradox that typifies this new view of the world is that we are all one but we are all separate. Ego and the old paradigm believe in separation and individuation. A holistic culture embraces the paradox of separation and togetherness, division and intimacy. This is the dance of outer self and inner self, ego and soul, matter and spirit and it is one of the many lessons of our physical presence. We are all one yet we are all unique individuals.

In a physical world, being separate and being one are seen as a duality, two opposing aspects. In a metaphysical world, separation and unity are part of each other. Each can exist together and at the same time and although they seem contradictory, they are still true.

We seek to become one and we seek to stay individual. In this way, relationships help us learn how to do both things. In every relationship there is the dance between intimacy and individuality. Within us, this is mirrored by the dance between our physical self – the body and the mind, and our metaphysical self – our soul. We are separate and we are together.

A metaphysical culture embraces paradox because paradox teaches us more about holism and more about ourselves.

3. Vocabulary

At present, much of our language is based upon the left brain and on mechanistic beliefs. When we try to describe a new belief system using the language of the old belief system we run into problems. We need to develop the language as we go and be aware that some of our problems are due to the meanings of words as they have been used over the past few hundred years.

Other problems are encountered because the definitions of many words aren't always agreed upon. Sometimes this is because there are a few quite different meanings given for one word.

One of my friends and I used to have difficulties and I could never work out why until one day, I realised that our definition of friendship differed dramatically. Often it is the same in intimate relationships where one partner has one set of ideas about the relationship and the other has their own.

Usually the difference lies in what beliefs each of us holds. While 'friendship' and 'relationship' are just words, they also stand for concepts. These concepts are made up of content and process so that each of us holds very specific sets of beliefs. Any word that stands for any type of relationship can be interpreted quite differently between people or communities.

The language of holism seeks to give better definition to such words and concepts. The defining of such things is part of the relationship and it cannot be overlooked. Disagreements between people and communities and countries need to be seen as partly related to the differences in how we define words and concepts.

Fundamental to resolving different beliefs and definitions is the ability to recognise these differences and address them honestly.

While culture is partly about language and ideas, the other two fundamental aspects of Western culture are science and religion. The next chapter deals with science and the change in paradigms between the old world view and a new holistic world view.

The third chapter in this part looks at religion and at what a holistic religious view might be like.

Two - The Science of Holism

Before I begin this chapter, let me state that I do not consider myself an expert in scientific theory. What follows is a simplified idea of how holism can be just as scientifically based as our old mechanistic world view. Again, it depends upon our definition of the word 'science'.

'Science' apparently derives from the Latin *scientia*, which means having knowledge, or its present participle *scire*, meaning to know. As we have already seen, knowledge is not an absolute thing, it is related to what we perceive, which is related to what we believe. I will define science as 'the current state of knowledge'.

At present, the current state of knowledge in the biological sciences (including medicine) is lagging behind the physical sciences.

Over the past few hundred years, science (both physical and biological) has been based upon mechanistic and physically orientated beliefs and laws. These laws of science came about during the scientific revolution, through changes in the sixteenth and seventeenth centuries. I won't go into detail about these changes but they were brought about by brilliant new theories and different ways of looking at the world.

There was a major change in world view from the earth being thought of as at the centre of the universe to a planet in a minor part of the universe (Copernicus and Galileo). Galileo also produced an empirical and mathematical approach to describing nature, while Bacon developed the method of scientific inductive reasoning. Descartes (famous for 'Cogito, ergo sum') introduced analytical thinking and deductive reasoning, the idea of the mind and body as separate and of life like a machine.[19] Isaac Newton brought these ideas and beliefs together and produced a theory of the world based upon a mechanistic view of nature (Mathematical Principles of Natural Philosophy). Newtonian physics is based upon the principle that laws and rules that are rationally understood govern the universe.

While some of these beliefs were modified over the centuries, scientists operated (and many continue to operate) under the belief that this mechanistic world view was truth, that everything could be (and needed to be) explained rationally.

In 1900, quantum mechanics was born and physicists began to question the validity of Newtonian physics and the mechanistic world view. Quantum mechanics is the study of quanta – very small things – and their behaviour or motion. As smaller and smaller particles of matter were discovered, it became apparent that sub-atomic particles and their movement or behaviour could not be explained rationally.

Many people were involved in the birth and growth of quantum mechanics. Max Planck was probably the father, with his discovery in 1900 of 'quanta', although Albert Einstein[20] was probably the stepfather with his groundbreaking work that cut across many areas.

In 1905, Einstein published five papers that revolutionised the science of physics. The three main ones were to do with the special theory of relativity, the quantum theory of radiation and a theory of Brownian movement. His ideas and the work of numerous

---

19   I have not read their full works but apparently Descartes in particular had a much broader view of the world than we now give him credit for. Nevertheless we take the parts we want and historically we look back and attribute the birth of the mechanistic world view to these men and their ideas.

20   This man was one of the greatest geniuses of our time, a truly brilliant thinker.

physicists and mathematicians led to a change in beliefs about the nature of physical reality. While not all scientists have embraced this change, it has led to a paradigm shift in thinking – another scientific revolution – a change from a mechanistic world view to a holistic or ecological world view.

This revolution in the physical sciences is due to three new ways of looking at the world – through relativity, quantum mechanics and chaos theory. All of them are interconnected. This is an oversimplification but these three areas help us understand how the new holistic world view is so different from the old mechanistic world view. I don't claim to understand everything to do with relativity, quantum mechanics and chaos theory but what I take from these areas are two main things. The first is that they provide a new view of reality (in contrast to the old mechanistic Newtonian Cartesian world view). The second is that this new view is in fact a very old view, an Eastern view of reality. In many ways, the Western world has begun to prove scientifically what Eastern traditions have long known.

For a far better description of these areas than I can give, I recommend you read one of the numerous books on the subject. The Dancing Wu Li Masters by Gary Zukav, The Elegant Universe by Brian Greene, The Turning Point by Fritjof Capra, and Chaos by James Gleick.[21]

Relativity

Like many scientists before him, Einstein was a genius because he was able to see beyond the beliefs of his time. He was not restricted by absolute ideas of reality but able to imagine other possibilities.

---

21   See Bibliography for details.

His special theory of relativity, which he published in 1905, was a product of his ability to go beyond the beliefs of his day. Some years before, various experiments had demonstrated that the speed of light was a constant (186,000 miles/second). This contradicted the Newtonian belief (actually Galilean) that the speed of anything was relative to something else. If we walk at six kilometres/hour and our friend runs at 10 kilometres/hour then our friend is effectively going at four kilometres/hour relative to us. In this way if light is travelling at 186,000 miles/second and we are travelling at 100,000 miles/second then the light should only be going at 86,000 miles/second relative to us. Experimentally, physicists discovered that no matter how fast we are going light is still travelling at 186,000 miles/second relative to us.

While many theorists tried to work out what was going wrong with the experiments, Einstein tried to work out what was wrong with the theory. He postulated that the speed of light is actually constant but that the tools we use to measure speed (distance over time) are altered the faster they travel. So as speeds increase, time slows (the clocks actually go slower and the length of objects contract in the direction of travel), in other words, there is no such thing as absolute time. If we were to travel through space for a year at high speed, when we returned to earth we would not have aged as much as those left behind.

Einstein's special theory of relativity views space and time as space-time, an inseparable continuum.[22]

We live in a four-dimensional reality (depth, width, length, time) but we perceive it as three dimensional (depth, width, length) travelling forward (time). What we perceive, that everything moves forward with time, may not really be how it is.

22   A continuum is something that cannot be broken down into parts. So space-time as a continuum cannot be broken down into space and time.

The other more famous part of Einstein's special theory of relativity is the equation E=mc squared. Energy equals mass multiplied by the speed of light squared (this is very fast). What this means is that matter and energy are not two separate things. In many ways, there is also a mass-energy continuum. While it was once thought that the universe was made up of a finite amount of mass and a finite amount of energy (law of conservation), Einstein's discovery meant that the universe is now thought to have a finite amount of mass-energy. Mass can move to energy and energy can move to mass but there is a finite amount of mass-energy.[23]

Einstein's special theory of relativity (and the research that confirmed it all) proved that our previous assumptions were limited. Our ideas about the nature of reality were limited.

Quantum mechanics

Quantum mechanics is the study of the smallest particles and their movement or behaviour.

From my reading, there are a number of discoveries in quantum mechanics and particle physics[24] that are particularly interesting and that lend weight to a holistic world view. However, what follows only touches the surface of an enormous subject.

Sub-atomic particles cannot be studied directly because they are too small. Each atom (which in Newtonian physics was thought to be the smallest particle of substance) is made up of sub-atomic particles. We have no way of seeing atoms, much less the parts of

---

23   While Einstein's discoveries have led to many advances and a greater understanding of 'reality', they also led to the development of the atomic bomb where uranium atoms undergo fission and release large amounts of energy. Mass becomes energy.

24   Quantum mechanics is the theory, particle physics comprise the practical experiments that back up the theory.

an atom. When physicists investigated their behaviour, what they discovered was that an atom is more space than matter.

Imagine that an atom is the size of a football stadium. If we can picture this then the nucleus of the atom, which is the largest material part of an atom, would be about as big as a grain of sand in the middle of the stadium. The electrons that orbit the nucleus would be as big as tiny dust particles and their orbits would include the whole stadium.

So most of the atom is space.

When physicists were able to study sub-atomic particles, they discovered that even these 'things' (the grain of sand that is the nucleus and the dust particle electrons that orbit the nucleus) were not really matter.

As scientists studied the behaviour of sub-atomic particles, they discovered that the particles could not be measured as things that were moving. They could only be measured as things or as movement. The particle exhibits a wave-like pattern that is dancing between mass (thing) and energy (movement). (If you have been following any of this you will realise that this is what Einstein had predicted in his E=mc squared equation – energy and mass make up a continuum.)

Quantum physics demonstrated that the universe and its parts cannot be reduced to isolated particles or definite substance. The basic building blocks of matter are not building blocks at all – rather they are energy connections. These energy connections do not operate in a logical manner. Instead, they operate according to probabilities.

When studying a sub-atomic particle, for example a photon, quantum physics can determine the probability of an outcome but not the actual outcome.

Quantum physics talks about probabilities of events occurring, but as matter is broken down into smaller and smaller units, it seems that the connections between particles are as important as the particles themselves.

Chaos

Relativity and quantum physics made scientists rethink their approach. The old mechanistic Newtonian and Cartesian rules no longer held true for all systems, but they still were no closer to being able to describe how systems work. They had rejected the old idea of being able to reduce a system into its parts to discover how the system worked, but they were left with the equally mysterious knowledge that the particles within a system were somehow affected by the system as a whole.

In the 1970s physicists, mathematicians and even some biologists began to turn their attention to the behaviour of systems. Chaos is the science of the global nature of systems, and the global nature of systems is that they operate via non-linear processes. These processes are unpredictable, through the lens of our current knowledge, yet they still move towards order. The chaotic system moves towards order. Non-linear processes are said to be irrational; this means they cannot be described in a rational logical way and to the left brain they seem like nonsense. Einstein showed that what seems like nonsense to the logical left brain could often be proven a better version of reality with time.

I have already written about chaos and non-linear processes in earlier chapters so I won't go into more detail here. Chaos theory turned the attention away from the content of life and the universe towards the process. The discoveries of quantum physics, that the smallest particles in life were both matter and energy (substance and wave motion), were mirrored in the finding that both content and process comprise part of larger systems. While the mechanistic view of the world separated content from process and concentrated on linear processes, the new holistic view takes into account content and process (linear and non-linear) and views these two parts as inseparable.

Holistic Laws

The word holism simply refers to the whole thing – everything. Physical and spiritual, content and process and the connections between two seemingly separate ideas come together in this word. Yet holism is defined as much as anything by its mysterious nature. In mechanistic and logical terms, it is indefinable. It is not a fixed thing so much as an ever-changing system. Our previous world view led us to believe that with enough knowledge we could know something. The holistic view is that things are not knowable in a purely rational way.

Mechanistic science is largely content based, that is, it relies upon analysing the content of a system to draw conclusions. It draws upon the linear process but often fails to see the connections between content and process. Holistic science is both content and process based. In holistic science, both the content and the process are important and they cannot be seen as separate things because even they are connected.

Holism has at its basis the idea that everything is connected to everything else in ways that we cannot yet define, or cannot understand with our left brain. The connections are energetic in nature but they do not always behave according to the currently known laws of physics. For example, some of the connections might operate faster than the speed of light.

Holism implies a system that is connected to other systems and is in a constant state of movement or change. The movement is towards integration, order and further growth or expansion.

In human terms, therefore, each human is part of a larger system and is connected to the other parts of the larger system. In fact, a human cannot be separated in real terms from the other parts. Our ideas of each human being as a separate thing is an approximation. We are only approximately separate in physical terms. In metaphysical or energetic terms, we are not separate from anything else in the system.

Each human in the larger system is in a constant state of motion, on several levels. At the sub-atomic level, there is more space than particle and our particles are constantly moving between matter and energy. At this level, we aren't technically substance. Our particles are like waves whose motion is ruled not by fate but by probabilities. The future of these particles is always only a probable future and it can change at any time.

At the microscopic level, we are made up of millions of cells, each a system in itself yet each not separate from the other cells. Each communicates with the others in ways we still don't understand. Each cell moves through its life cycle so that over a number of years none of the original cells is still alive. There is constant movement – birth, life, death, birth, life, death, birth, life... This is part of our internal system that determines our physical presence.

Then there is our metaphysical self whose movement is no less complex. This self in our human form is inseparable from our physical self. We can try and pay attention only to our physical self or only to our spiritual self, but this approach reflects our tendency towards separation. These selves are not separable in this physical life, although at physical death they will separate. In holistic terms, a human is an ever-changing system connected to every other system and a part of every other system. Within the human system, the two seemingly separate parts are not separate. Physical and spiritual are part of each other. Content and process are part of each other.

On a sub-atomic level, the particles have no predictable future, only probable or most likely futures. On a systems level the process of chaos carries this same unpredictability. The process of chaos does result in order; however, we have no way of knowing what that order will be. While we may have an idea of the probable future this is only a probability, not a predetermined outcome.

We still do not know in scientific terms what drives this process and what determines the outcome. But not knowing does not stop us living and this is what holism demands of a system – that it follow the process of life. The only constant in a holistic system is change; movement is inherent within the system.

It seems to me that growth is the change that the human system is designed for or is working towards, and that this growth is in all dimensions (physical and spiritual). It is also connected to the growth of everything else in the system. Growth of humans is dependent upon multiple factors within the system, which in logical terms can never be defined. However, growth occurs best when the system is well integrated and therefore in balance, although not in the linear sense of balance.

Holistic reality

Holistic reality is not a stable definable thing; it is dynamic and always moving. It is like the Taoist concept of the dynamic interplay between yin and yang – there is always movement between these two phases as they try to reach a balance, however the balance is never reached because part of the balance is the movement between the two phases.

We seek a balance between intellect and intuition, feelings and physical sensing, being and doing, receiving and giving, the right side and the left side, spirit and physical manifestation. The balance is always moving and the system is never completely still. Balance in this sense is not linear as on a scale. It is an integration of our parts, but the degree of integration is always moving like a dance.

We look at the tiny atom and see a particle or a wave, depending on how we look. We look at a human and see substance or change, depending on how we look. This is the paradox of holism – that everything is substance and movement, mass and energy, but neither can be defined separately. As humans, we are both mass and energy, physical and spiritual but these two parts cannot be separated and within each part exists part of the other.

Whenever we try to define holism, we go around in circles because we are trying to define a right-brain idea in left-brain language. We never fully encapsulate it, but the more we try the closer we get until at some point we will intuitively understand what it means. This is the paradox of holism for the traditional scientist and the traditional doctor – it cannot be defined in left-brain terms, we cannot understand holism with our left-brain processes.

THREE - THE RELIGION OF HOLISM

In this chapter we are faced with the age-old conundrum – is there a God? If so, whose God is the right one?

The answer to these questions lies in our belief about truth. Our left brain believes there is a yes or no answer to the question. If the answer is yes there is a god, then there must be a right one and therefore many wrong ones. Our soul and our right brain believe there is not one correct answer to the question and that the answer will continually change depending upon our level of consciousness and knowledge. What we believe to be truth is simply a belief, not a fact. The truths we believe in this century are different from the truths we believed in last century.

How do these changes in beliefs come about? Why?

At the heart of all life is the principle of growth. Growth is essentially the never-ending process of creation.

In the physical world, most physical growth concerns itself with the creation of matter. A plant grows and in doing so creates more plant material – stems, roots, leaves, seeds, fruit. The cycle of life ensures that the growth of the plant leads to the production of fertile seed so that even if the plant dies, the genetic material continues to grow, produce and create more plants. But even the growth of the plant is not solely about the production of seed. All the physical material produced by the plant – stem, roots, leaves, flowers, and seeds – are also part of a larger system that provides food and shelter for many animals and other plants, and oxygen and other gases that help maintain the system we call earth.

Humans too exhibit amazing physical growth in their early years as they mature to the stage where they are able to reproduce. But we also grow intellectually, emotionally and intuitively. These aspects of our self grow and expand – or not, depending on whether or not we are to open to growth and expansion.

Our growth as souls is towards growth in consciousness. This occurs as we become more aware of who we really are. We begin to bring to our conscious awareness those parts of ourselves that have previously been unconscious.

This happens throughout our lives.

We move from toddlers ruled by fantasy and imagination to children who begin to see things in a linear way and go on to develop concrete rational thinking. During this time we are developing physically at a fast pace. Our emotional and intuitional growth often take a back seat until around adolescence, they begin to reassert their needs.

As our consciousness expands in adolescence, we begin to define ourselves more in relationship to other people (non-family members). We may rebel against our parents and society but typically we find some type of group to which we primarily relate and feel we belong. This stage of development mirrors a conventional (or fundamental) religious world view.

As we become adults (usually during the process of leaving home), we begin to see ourselves as more defined individuals in our own right. We begin to reflect on who we are, separate from our relationships. The power of the rational mind takes centre stage.

In this stage, we are egocentric but because we are aware that relationships with other people are important, part of our concerns centre around our relationships and how they affect us. This stage is typical of a humanistic world view. This view largely rules science and in particular medicine, although there is still a large section of Western society that holds conventional religious beliefs.

As we mature as adults, we often develop a growing awareness of our inner self. We become conscious of this deeper level of self – not just the ego voice in our head but an inner self. This stage typically occurs from the age of thirty onwards but it may not occur at all. Some people may live their whole adult lives with a conventional religious or a humanistic world view.

As we become aware of our inner self, we also become aware that we are part of something bigger and that it is part of us. Our soul is always pushing us to a greater awareness. Growth in consciousness and the integration of our spiritual and physical aspects continues throughout our life. As we approach death, our consciousness continues to expand and we gradually leave the physical dimensions.

At each stage, we can only see from the viewpoint of our current state of consciousness and our previous stages. We cannot see or understand a world view or stage of consciousness that is more advanced than, or beyond, our own.

We have trouble remembering what we believed when we were toddlers and children but usually we clearly remember our previous stage of development. We often yearn for those simpler times. Once we see the next stage and our awareness grows, it is almost impossible to go backwards. We may try because some part of us seeks to revisit the safety and simplicity of previous stages. It is simpler to believe that I am just the voice in my head and that I can control life through rational thought processes and the power of the mind.

Society mirrors this dilemma. Politicians and religious leaders are always reminiscing about the good old days and seeking to return society to former times, where former beliefs and values were more easily defined and appeared to be stable. But growth and expansion are what the soul seeks and spiritual growth is about movement and change.

While we might think we wish for the simplicity of childhood with its structure and illusions of safety and security, what our inner selves wish for is to continue growing. When we reach a certain age and think we can stop learning, we can be sure our inner self, our soul, will not be quiet. Things will happen to get us moving. Soul and spirit will shake things up a little, or a lot. The cycles of life cannot be ignored. The passages we go through in our physical lives continue right up until we die. This brings us back to the original question – is there a god? If so, whose god is the right one?

First, we need to define the question. Do we mean a personal god as defined by many religions, or a metaphorical god?

Holistically, God cannot be separate from everything else, so God is both personal and metaphorical. But the image of a god who sits in heaven in judgement on us all is a remnant of a patriarchal flat world. None of us can answer the question of God, but we do know that what we think is truth is only ever a belief about truth. We also know that each of us is striving to expand our awareness, which includes an awareness of the unifying force behind our existence. By definition, such a unifying force would be completely beyond our comprehension because it would exist beyond this physical world. All of our attempts at defining such a unifying force (God) are doomed to failure simply because we are defining something using our physical terms of reference. That does not mean we should stop trying. The way to understand such a unifying force is first to understand ourselves, because ultimately part of each of us is this unifying power.

This unifying power is what I have previously referred to as spirit but what many people might call God. I do not view spirit as a separate being. Rather, spirit is within each of us and is throughout everything. We are part of it and it is part of us. We cannot be separated because we are the same, and therefore we are all connected to everything else by this sameness. In a sense, part of me is the same as part of you is the same as part of everyone else. This is our connection, this is spirit, this is the unifying force.

A mystical experience of any kind puts us in touch with this sameness, this oneness. We can have such a mystical experience whatever our stage of development or level of consciousness.

If we have a conventional religious world view, we might experience this in a religious setting such as a church service and label it 'the presence of the holy spirit'.

People with a humanistic world view might more often experience this through nature or community or in relationships and label it 'communing with nature' or 'intimacy'.

With a holistic world view we realise that the mystical experience might be available to us all the time if we could learn how. This is the essence of holism, which is to learn how to live from our souls and thereby allow spirit to flow through us.

The mystic seeks to discover the mystery behind the universe or spirit but because part of us is the same as the universe, we are really seeking to discover ourselves. As we discover more about ourselves, we discover more about the universe.

Science seeks to increase our knowledge of the physical world and religions seek to increase our understanding of the spiritual world.

Religions are also one way we attempt to categorise and exert control over spirit or God – often through prayer, worship or ritual.

Holism doesn't have a religion in the conventional sense of the word. Its religion is its inclusion of spirit in the whole of life. In that sense it returns to a similar view held by traditional cultures, but there is a difference. The difference is in the conscious awareness of the self as part of the whole.

I believe we might categorise human evolution, or growth of consciousness, in four stages. This is not to say that this is a linear process. It may be a spiral or a cycle. It may be non-linear. But for an explanation of how we might live whole lives it helps to understand where we are in relation to these four stages. Usually, we are across a few of the stages rather than being solidly in any one stage (although some of us are there too).

The first stage I would call unconscious holism.[25] This is typical of most traditional cultures where people are part of the system they live in and act in ways that support the system. They live within a greater system in harmony – the physical and the spiritual are intertwined and this is simply how life is. There is not a conscious awareness of this in most of these people and their world view is limited to their tribe or a collection of tribes.

As various tribes and cultures begin to mix, the world view changes to one of unconscious duality. 'Us' and 'them' are seen as different and the system begins to become more polarised. The notion of physical and spiritual as separate rather than connected

25   I came across a variation of these terms in Alan Oken's book, Astrology for the Soul. He talks about three stages – unconscious unity, conscious duality and conscious unity. I have borrowed from his ideas.

takes shape, albeit at an unconscious level. Normal everyday life and spiritual (now religious) life become separate. The world is seen in terms of good and bad, us and them, right and wrong. This is typical of many fundamental religions and mechanistic scientists. This stage I would call unconscious duality. We are not conscious that the categories of right and wrong, the dualisms that govern life, are actually just beliefs about reality.

Gradually the wheel turns and people become conscious of this duality so that the physical and the spiritual are seen as part of the dual nature of life. In this stage, people begin to try to balance the physical and spiritual sides of life in a conscious manner. Conscious duality. This stage is all about finding balance between the various seemingly opposing aspects of our self.

This leads to conscious holism, which is a conscious effort to become whole, to bring the physical and spiritual aspects back into harmony: to live as part of the larger system, to know that we are part of God, or the divine, or the unifying force of spirit, and that we have our own unique part to play in creating a better system. We become conscious that spirit and matter are the same and we learn how to live whole lives consciously. We manifest our own unique bit of spirit in the physical world.

Once we get expert at being whole, the process possibly becomes unconscious, we return to unconscious holism and the cycle continues. With each cycle, the circle expands to include a larger system: from the tribe, to the country, to earth and then beyond.

Now that we have a bit of the theory behind us, in Part four we look at the process behind becoming more conscious of our holistic nature.

HOLISTIC MEDICINE

Long, long ago before anyone remembers, people lived in complete harmony with themselves, each other, all the animals, birds, fish, crawling creatures, all the planet, and the Great Mystery of the all. This was a time of easy blissful living, and life was happy and serene.

As time went on, the humans began to forget what they knew. They gradually became selfish and self-centred and started to believe that they were above creation and better than the rest of creation. They pulled themselves out of oneness and established hierarchy, not only setting themselves apart, they set themselves above.

During those times, there were elders in the tribe who had been given the responsibility of keeping and protecting the wisdom of the tribe. Because they were so wise and so old, they had the perspective to see what had been and what was happening, and they became greatly concerned. They called a meeting of all the elders who were responsible for the wisdom of the tribe and spent many long days and nights discussing what they should do.

'The people are becoming like children,' one said. 'They are selfish and self-centred. They only think of themselves and abuse what the creator gives them.'

'They abuse our Mother, the earth, and do not recognise that everything we have, our food, our clothing, our shelter comes from her,' another added.

'They have forgotten that they are spiritual beings and all is spiritual,' confided another, and they talked long days and long nights.

At last the elders decided that the people had become so lost and their minds and hearts so distorted that they could no longer be trusted with the spiritual wisdom that had sustained the people for so long. Since they were the guardians of the wisdom, they were determined that it would not be abused, and vowed to protect it at all costs. Therefore the elders decided to gather up all the wisdom and tie it in a big bundle and hide it.

'Where shall we hide it so that they won't find it until they are ready?' an old woman asked. 'We must pray and think on this.' They all agreed. Again, they devoted several days and nights fasting and praying about their next steps.

'When they sat down together, the elder asked, 'Have we come upon a solution?'

'I know,' said one. 'There is a tall mountain far off in the forest and within that mountain there is a deep hidden cave no one knows about. Let us take the bundle of wisdom, dig a big hole far back in the cave, and bury it deep underground. They'll never find it there.'

The elders sat silent for a while and pondered this possibility.

'They are tricky these people. They are always snooping around and looking into everything. Sooner or later they are sure to find the cave and they will start digging around and find it.'

Slowly they let this information sink in, and then sadly, they all agreed. 'You're right! They do go everywhere and get into everything.'

Saddened they sat a while longer.

'I know!" said another. 'I know a very, very deep lake. We do not even know the bottom. Let's wrap it up very carefully and sink it way, way down in the lake. They'll never find it there.'

Initially the elders felt hopeful with this solution as they were weary and wanted to know what to do. Yet they also knew that this was a grave matter and they had an important responsibility. Slowly each came to know that the lake was not an answer.

'No, they like to fish. Sooner or later someone would hook it and pull it up. We can't do that.'

Again the elders sat motionless for what seemed like an eternity.

Then very slowly an old woman elder, the oldest among them spoke. "I know what we must do,' she said carefully speaking with wisdom and authority.

'We will hide it inside of them, they will never look there.'

And they all knew...they had their answer.

Traditional Native American story

ONE - A DIFFERENT WORLD VIEW

Holistic medicine is a different world view because at its core is the belief that we can all heal ourselves. This healing is not, however, just on a physical level but on a physical and spiritual level. The two aspects both need healing in order to live whole lives. Holistic medicine is therefore about helping people learn how to heal themselves.

I believe we each have the ability to heal ourselves. I believe the reason we are not healthy is because we are not living our own life. We are living a life that we think we should live or that someone else thinks we should live. We live this life because we were never taught to pay attention to our own self.

We all have diseases and illnesses; they are a large part of modern life.

Dis–ease. Not at ease.

We aren't at ease with our whole self. Most of us live lives that we are not at ease with and this makes us sick. Physical illness, mental illness, emotional illness, spiritual illness.

The reason we have any illness is because we need it on some level. If we can fulfil that need in other healthier ways, we can heal our illnesses.

The human system is capable of healing itself. If you cut your finger with a knife the body will heal itself. If you have a disease or illness, the body is capable of healing that illness but it has to be given the right conditions. Healing our illness is about giving our body the opportunity to heal by giving it the right conditions to bring about healing.

The first point to remember, however, is that for some reason we need this illness or disease. This is a different approach to conventional medicine, which always seeks to be rid of the disease. Holistic medicine views disease as a way to heal our fragmentation, move into wholeness, discover who we really are and what we have come here to do.

Illness and diseases have many messages for us. When I talk about illness and disease, I include emotional and spiritual crises that affect our wellbeing.

Sometimes, it is soul's way of bringing us to a greater awareness of who we really are and of what is important for our lives.

Sometimes, disease is the body's way of bringing our attention to things we have been ignoring.

Sometimes, a chronic illness is our system's attempt to keep us in balance.

Often, illness brings us back to an understanding of how we need to look after ourselves better, or how we need to look after the systems (family, community, society, earth) better so that the world we live in is healthy and supports our health.

Ultimately, all illness is about fulfilling our needs. When we forget that we need to look after ourselves, we get sick. This applies on many levels. We cannot just look after our physical needs and expect to be healthy. We have to also become aware of our spiritual needs and learn how to fulfil them.

In simple terms, all diseases have both a physical and a spiritual component. The physical component is about how we are not fulfilling our physical needs and the spiritual component is about how we are not fulfilling our spiritual needs. Paradoxically, the illness or disease helps us fulfil the needs that we are not aware of. If we become aware of these needs, we can learn how to heal ourselves by fulfilling them in other ways.

At the same time, illness is a much more complex process. It is seldom linear, that is, there is seldom a direct cause and effect relationship. We might look at obesity and say that the cause is eating too much of the wrong food or doing too little exercise, but the meaning behind obesity is multifactorial. It is a complex process that the human system has developed in order to get its needs met. It is likely that the 'cause' of obesity in one person is quite different from the cause in another.

If we take obesity as an example, we can look at it from a purely physical perspective. It is true that the person is eating too much and doing too little. Their intake (energy in) is higher than their output (energy expended) so the extra energy is stored as weight. The answer to weight loss from this perspective is simple – eat less, do more.

If we look at it from a purely spiritual perspective, we might view obesity as a form of protection – insulating oneself from the world or in some people, a need for grounding. Spiritual interpretation of illness is a look at the deeper issues – what does the obesity give us?

Holistic medicine looks at any disease or symptom from both these points of view. What is the physical perspective? What is the spiritual perspective? Then it seeks to help the patient learn how to fulfil those needs in ways that are more useful.

The illness helps us uncover more about who we really are and what we need in order to be whole people. I like to think the human system is clever and that if we get out of our own way we can heal ourselves. Trouble is, we can't stop meddling in our own natural process of healing. We have trouble just letting things be. We have trouble supporting our body to heal because this is harder than finding a quick fix. We like to control things and we dislike illness because it interferes with our plans. However, most of our plans are products of our left brain and Western society. These plans are not always in line with what our inner self, our soul, has in mind. Illness is about paying better attention to our inner self and the needs of our physical and spiritual halves.

Things become even more complex when we consider that we are not just half-physical, half-spiritual. We are also made up of our four basic elements (earth, fire, water, air). Each element has needs of its own and we are unconsciously trying to find a way to balance the needs of all our parts.

A further level of complexity is that we are part of a larger system. The people we have relationships with, the community we live in, the earth as a whole, all these affect us via our etheric connections. We need to pay these some attention as well.

The other level of complexity is that of time. We live in a world where processes are important. Life is always moving. There are cycles that we are part of – day and night, seasons, years, lifetimes.

To look at an illness from a holistic perspective is an immensely complex task.

From a holistic perspective, we look at the person on several levels in order to work out how they can maximise their healing.

1. Balance. We look at the balance of our four basic elements – fire, water, air, and earth.

2. Harmony. We look at our connections (ether) – connection to our inner spiritual self, connection to other people, connection to the larger system of earth.

3. Living the cycles. We look at the cycles and processes that we are living.

First, let's look at some guidelines behind holistic healing.

TWO - HEALING OURSELVES

⌒‿⌒

This chapter is about bringing it together. When we learn what it is to live our whole life, we become the person we are meant to be. We stop being the person we think we should be and start just being ourselves.

When we can be ourselves, we are living whole lives. It may not be the life you envisaged, or that you had planned, or that your family and friends thought you should live, or the life that society had mapped out for you. It is your life. Living the life you were meant to live is what we all came here to do.

Most of us learn how to live our life through the process of living. Realistically, we are always learning more about ourselves and about the system in which we live. But we get to a stage in our life where we become more comfortable simply to be ourselves. We become aware when we are not being ourselves and not living whole lives.

There are several general principles or guidelines that we need to consider when we are talking about healing from a holistic perspective.

Principle 1 – Question all the rules

A rule is a guideline that has been prescribed by someone. Someone else has thought up most of the rules we live by but we blindly follow them. We often don't even think to question them. We often follow other people's beliefs and rules simply because we haven't even thought about whether they are right or not.

As children, we don't learn to question things enough. We are taught that some things just are and that we should accept that. Part of growing up and taking responsibility for our own lives is that we question the rules of society that don't feel right to us. We decide not to live according to the rules that don't make sense.

A basic assumption of holism is that we have a right to live in a way that makes sense to us as a unique individual. We have a choice about how we live our lives.

Most of us are not aware that we are living by rules that someone else has decided on, or that our beliefs about the nature of things may be wrong. This is why it helps us to become conscious of these things. The easiest way to become more conscious is to question all the rules. To question them, we have to become aware of them.

What we are questioning is the basic belief system that we live by. This belief system is not truth but we think that it is. The first principle of holistic healing is to question all our rules and belief systems.

Principle 2 – Trust yourself

The second principle of holistic healing is that we need to learn how to trust ourselves. We need to trust that we know what is best for us. We have a responsibility to get our needs met but we are learning how to trust that we know what these needs are.

As we pay better attention to our elements and begin to use our intuitive and emotional abilities better, we learn that we have the answers to our own problems. We learn that we know what is best for us in any given situation. This is a hard thing to re-learn because we have been taught not to trust ourselves.

But we try. We try to trust that we know which decision is best and so we make a decision. We try to trust that the situation we are in is for our own growth and learning so we stop fighting and let things happen naturally. We try to trust that the small inner voice is telling us the truth even when it seems out of step with the rest of the world, or our community, or our family.

The only way we can demonstrate trust in ourselves is by doing the things we need to do.

We all have various needs and some of these seem to be competing with each other. We have a need to feel safe and secure but we also have a need to take risks. We have a need to be connected to other people but we also have a need for isolation. We need rest but we also need work and play. We need to give love and receive love. We need to do things that manifest our uniqueness in the physical world.

We need certain things in our life to be happy and healthy and whole. We also want certain things. A need, however, is much more important to our wholeness than a want. Western society emphasises fulfilment of desires. It tries to tell us that we can all have anything we want. Maybe we can if we don't care about the rest of the system.

On earth, certain resources are limited. This is the restriction of physical manifestation. If we go after everything we want then it is likely that other parts of the system will suffer. Some other people won't have enough, animals will have nowhere to live and the planet will not be able to sustain our rampant consumption.

As part of our healing, we are also learning about how we fit into the larger system. We fit in by being ourselves. To be ourselves we have to get our needs fulfilled and we have to play our part in helping other people fulfil their needs. We have to be conscious of the whole system, and of how what we do affects the health of the system. If we use up all of earth's resources and pollute the land and sea and air then we need to be aware that this will have negative effects on the earth and therefore on us. We cannot be whole and healthy in isolation. We can only be whole and healthy when the system is whole and healthy.

As part of the system, we have a two-fold responsibility.

We have a responsibility to our self.

We have a responsibility to the system that we are part of.

As we become more aware of the lack of wholeness in our self, we become more aware of the lack of wholeness in the system. Our communities are not whole, our society is not whole, the earth is not whole. The paradox of course is that we are all whole. It's just that we aren't fully aware of this, so we are driven by forces that seem not to be part of us.

When I talk about not being whole, I really mean that we aren't aware of our whole self. This means that the systems we are part of are not aware either because we are the part of the system with the highest consciousness. Currently, we lack awareness that we are part of larger systems and that we are partly responsible for their wellbeing. We are like bacteria on the human body that have no idea of the part they play in the larger system. We, as humans, can become conscious of the part we play in the system.

Principle 3 – Trust the process of life

Life will follow its natural process no matter what we do. The cycles of life and the processes that drive the cycles will occur irrespective of our actions. It is these processes and cycles that bring about growth and transformation. We trust that within us we have the wisdom to get through the other side of the process transformed. We don't know what we will transform into, soul doesn't know, spirit doesn't know because the process never leads to a set outcome. That is its beauty of course – the outcome is unpredictable.

If we wanted a crop of perfect corn, we would take the seed of what we consider to be perfect corn and grow the crop. We might genetically engineer the corn to make it perfect and ensure that all the seeds of the corn are the same as the seeds of the parent corn. We know that our crop will always be the same. We have reached what we consider to be perfection.

We have, however, lost all the potential. If we make a mistake and forget one important thing, like resistance to an unforeseen attack by viruses, then the seed has reached the end of the road. All our corn was perfect (or so we thought) but now it's all dead.

Our knowledge or our level of awareness therefore always limits our belief about perfection. Perfection is a left-brain concept. We seek perfection when we might be better seeking greater potential. The corn that was seemingly perfect turns out to have too little potential for change. The beauty of humans is that we have unlimited potential for change and transformation.

The inherent beauty of nature lies not only in what exists right now but also in the potential that exists. That potential is within all of us and the process of life simply helps us find our potential. If we live by linear rules then we fail to take advantage of the greatest gift we have, which is allowing the process of life to occur within us and thereby reach our potential.

I can't pretend to understand exactly how it all works but I have that potential. All of us have potential for things we never thought possible. Largely we never thought they were possible because we never let the possibility enter our conscious awareness.

Well, let it enter now.

The potential that exists within your inner self (your whole being) is as great as anyone else's.

So we take our first step. We decide to trust our self and follow the process of life to see where it takes us. Effectively, we give up the idea of control. Controlling our life is one of our limited beliefs, it is an illusion.

Principle 4 – Let go of the desire to control the outcome – surrender control

This principle, which for me is always the hardest and one I need more lessons on, is to give up our ideas about outcomes.

This is the one step we must keep taking in order to heal. We give up the idea of controlling the outcome of the process that we are going through. We let go of our fixation about the end of the process and instead trust that the process will take us where we need to go.

We surrender control to our inner self. This is difficult because we are not fully conscious of this part of our self. It is like surrendering to a force greater than ourselves yet this greater power is also an essential part of us.

This giving up of control of outcomes is central to learning how to be our true selves. Our left brain and our ego desperately want to believe they can somehow control the outcome. We know from earlier in the book that this is a result of linear thinking and limited beliefs.

After my second child was born, I developed an acute lower back injury. I was flat on my back in hospital for a week and the muscle spasm was so painful that I couldn't even roll over to feed my baby. I had to give myself up to the illness and just follow along. It took three months before I felt almost back to normal and since then my lower back has given me intermittent pain.

At first, I tried to work out what had caused it and how to fix it but as time went on and no-one seemed to have any answers, I realised that it was a complex issue. I get back pain when I don't pay attention to my own needs, sometimes when I am angry about an issue but don't address it, sometimes because I do too much heavy work. It took me a long time to let go of the need to control the outcome. I wanted the back pain fixed. As I was able to shift and let go of the outcome I was able to understand how the back pain was always helping me become more aware of when I wasn't paying attention to my own needs.

This letting go of outcomes is the most difficult thing we have to do because it is completely against our old way of thinking. This is in fact one of the basics of the new paradigm, of holism itself.

The only outcome we are after is transformation into our wholeness. We might also avoid the belief that wholeness has within it the idea that there is an ending, that we become whole and then we are finished. We could say we are transforming into wholeness and that an aspect of wholeness is always further transformation.

Letting go of outcomes doesn't mean we have no idea about outcomes or hopes or goals. It means that we need to be sufficiently flexible to understand that the outcome we had fixed in our conscious mind is not always the outcome that supports our growth best.

Simply put, until we are fully in touch with our whole self we do not know ahead of time what outcome will turn out to be best for us. Our inner self may not even know this, yet our inner self knows that the way to reach the best outcome is to follow the natural process of our lives. This doesn't mean that we will never have the outcome we thought. Often we will because we are sufficiently conscious of our inner self to head in the right direction.

For a long time I had very fixed ideas about this book. I thought that the outcome would be that I would publish the book and make enough money to live on so that I could write more. The more I tried to make myself finish, the less the book came together.

I tried to put my intellect to work on how to finish the book and get it published, thinking that if I wrote at least a thousand words a day then I would finish it quicker. When the process was disrupted and I tried to control it, I had trouble writing a thousand words a day. When I forced myself to write them but didn't actually feel like writing, I usually had to delete them all anyway.

So instead, I gave myself up to the process and decided 'what will be will be'. I realised I had to let go of my fixed ideas about what the outcome would be, so I let go of the controlling and did what felt right. I spent time gardening and reading and a little time writing. That went on for about a week then suddenly without warning, I woke up and knew what I had to write next. In a few days, I wrote more than I had written in two months.

By letting go of our fixed ideas about outcomes and surrendering to the process of life, it always helps us follow the process better. As we follow the process, we begin to learn about our inner selves and about who we really are. We begin to let go of other people's ideas of who we are (parents, friends, family, teachers, society) and start to learn about our whole selves. We learn about what we need to do to heal ourselves.

Principle 5 – Pay attention (to your parts)

One of my daughters is learning how to drive. She gets frustrated that there are so many things to pay attention to – speed, checking mirrors, steering, other cars, the road, indicators, and more. This is part of the process of learning new skills – there are many things to learn. As we learn them, we eventually master the parts and then they become largely unconscious. We no longer have to pay so much attention to the parts. We learn how to do the whole thing (driving) without having to think about it.

What we are learning is how to live whole lives. We do this by learning about the parts of ourselves and the parts of the process. We pay attention to the parts of ourselves – the air, water, earth, fire, and ether – and we pay attention to the parts of the process.

Gradually we become more aware of our parts and of the process and we begin to live in a more holistic way. As we become more aware of our selves, we become aware of the part of our self that is wise and knows how to live. We might call this our inner self but really, it is our whole self. Yet because we are unaware of this wholeness, we believe this inner self to be a separate part.

So we begin to learn to pay attention to our inner self or inner guidance.

The combination of all our elements (which is uniquely our combination) tells us if things are right for us or not. If we feel good about something, we know it is right for us. If we feel bad about something, we know in some way it is not right for us. This feeling of good or bad is not simply an emotional state; it is a combination of feeling, intuition, our physical body, our logical thinking, and ether. I will refer to it as our inner guidance but it arises from our living whole. It is what we are learning about – how to be whole. We learn about it by living our lives.

This inner guidance isn't easy to categorise or explain because it is not a purely physical process. Sometimes we arrive at this 'feeling right' place quite suddenly – we just know that something is right for us. At other times, we need to spend time in contemplation or meditation to arrive at a place that feels right. Such places are not constant. What feels right today may not feel right in two months. But we need to develop this understanding of ourselves. We need to get better at identifying this 'it feels right for me' place and its opposing place – 'this feels wrong for me'.

Generally, our culture teaches us to discount these feelings and replace them with logic. Life teaches us that we live a more authentic life when we pay more attention to our inner selves than to the rules of the outer world.

When we are unwell, we need to pay closer attention to our inner guidance. It will let us know what we need to do in order to promote our natural healing abilities. Most of us aren't used to listening to ourselves when we get sick – we go to doctors so we can keep working. We don't pay attention to ourselves.

We will be getting clear messages through our physical body. If we are tired we need more rest, if we have no appetite we need to stop eating, if we feel like oranges we need to eat oranges. These messages are not difficult to interpret but our culture tells us to ignore them and just soldier on. We consequently get sicker because we don't pay attention. We push ourselves.

Illness is a time to stop and reflect. It is a time to give our bodies time to heal. It is a time to learn what we personally need in order to promote our healing.

The more serious the illness the more attention we need to pay.

Serious illness – cancer, strokes, heart attacks – usually get our attention. However, if we can learn how to pay attention before we get so sick then we are much less likely to have serious illness. The best preventative health is to learn how to pay attention to your body's needs and to get those needs fulfilled. There are no specific rules that I can give you that will keep you healthy because everyone's needs are different.

We can begin by paying attention to the messages from all our parts – earth, fire, water, air, and ether. As we become more aware of our whole self, we begin to have an increased awareness of our inner guidance. When we are not feeling so good we pay attention to this and reflect on what is out of balance. When we are feeling good, we reflect on this and do those things that promote continuing wellness.

Principle 6 – Take responsibility

Ultimately, we are responsible for ourselves. This means that we are responsible for determining what we need to be healthy and for trying to fulfil those needs.

At the same time, we are responsible for the health of the whole system. The responsibility we have to the whole system is that we be ourselves. We fulfil our needs and help others fulfil theirs. We don't have to help everyone, we only have to help those people we need to help. We have a responsibility to find this balance for ourselves. We learn how to say yes to our own needs and no to things we think we need but that actually make us less healthy. We learn how to say no to other people's demands that compromise our own health. We learn that helping others is what we are here for but that we can only do it in certain ways. We cannot be all things to all people.

We are the person who must take this responsibility for balancing our needs and the needs of the greater system or we will never be whole and healthy.

At one stage in my working life, I felt that I was letting the needs of my patients take precedence over my own needs. I could feel my energy being sucked out by so many patients needing so many things. I needed to remember I could not be all things to all people and that I must look after myself first. I felt like not working at all but my inner self somehow knew that was not what I needed to do. I felt drained by my work and it was because I was not being true to myself somehow in my work. I was working for a system that was not whole and I had let myself become like that system. I had lost myself again.

When we lose touch with our whole self, life feels wrong. In my case, I felt flat and drained. There was too little joy in my life, it was all seriousness and sickness. I knew something was terribly out of balance but I didn't know what to do about it. Unable to access my intuition, I went to see someone who might help me, a clairvoyant tarot reader. He told me work was killing me, or words to that effect. He told me I should get out. When I told him I had a contract until the end of the following year, he told me I needed to change my approach to work. I had to tap into my metaphysical side. So I had some answers to work with but I felt as if I was in the same place I had been many times before. Stuck in a job I didn't particularly enjoy. Yet this time was slightly different from before. Life goes in spirals and we often find ourselves in similar situations to those we have been in before. Can we use what we have learnt in the past to help us this time?

Principle 7 – Remember your lessons

If we are going to live consciously and pay attention, we always need to try to remember our previous lessons – those we are learning about our own healing, the lessons we become conscious of. We may need to unlearn some of the lessons that we had learnt unconsciously when we were at an earlier stage (see the next step).

We need to remember our new lessons because it often takes us a long while to learn something fully. The lessons are always building on the previous lesson but sometimes we get stuck because we drop back into old behaviours or limiting beliefs and forget what we know.

For all of us the previous lessons are different. The thing I usually forget is to trust the process. I battle the process. I pull it apart with my left brain and try to analyse it so I can solve the problem rationally. Then at some point I catch myself. 'You're doing it again,' I tell myself. 'Trust the process, let go of the outcome, pay attention to your feelings and intuition, stop thinking so much.' I could go on because there are many things I am learning about this process and it is taking me a long time! Each time I get stuck in chaos (and sometimes the chaos is only in my head), I try to remember what I have previously learnt and whether I am just stuck again because it is the same lesson.

It is like revision. We are often learning the same thing over and over until we get it. It becomes part of us. We no longer have to think how to walk or ride a bicycle or drive a car. Once we learn something on the physical level and master it, we can send it out of our consciousness – it becomes part of our new behaviour.

Our consciousness has a limited capacity. We can't be conscious of everything so as we master a lesson, we can then let it go and leave it up to our subconscious to remember it. When I am stuck in chaos, I review my recent lessons just to make sure this lesson isn't the same as the last one. Am I trusting the process? Have I let go of my need to try to control the outcome? Am I paying attention?

When I looked at how I was stuck in my work situation, I reviewed everything I had learnt about being stuck in this same place before. I thought I was trusting the process. I thought I was letting go of trying to control the outcome but I was not sure about that. I had not been paying myself enough attention. My life had been unbalanced for some time and I had not been able to address why I was so stuck. I thought I had not been paying my intuition or my feelings enough attention. But my inner guidance and intuition told me that what I was learning in this situation was probably a new lesson and that was why it was so hard. I kept trying to apply the old lessons when this was a new one.

While it is important to remember our old lessons, when we get really stuck in a chaotic problem it is usually because what we are trying to learn is a new lesson. We are being challenged by a new lesson that requires us to consider how we might change something about our lives. Often this means we need to let go of our past patterns of behaviour, or some other part of ourselves.

Principle 8 – Let go of the past

Much of what we have learnt in the more distant past is no longer useful. We learnt how to deal with things in a certain way but now we find that way was limited. We need to let go of those bits of our past that we no longer need. We can do this in various ways but essentially, it is about getting rid of our attachment to old stuff, to stuff we no longer need.

This is like dying. It is the stage of life where part of us has to die in order for new life to begin. We have to let go of our past patterns of behaviour because they do not support who we are becoming. Those patterns of behaviour were learnt in a different time and their usefulness was limited to that time.

We can consciously help ourselves to get rid of the past in a number of ways. It is good for us to get rid of everything that no longer nurtures us. All the physical stuff from our past that we no longer need, all the things we do that are not in line with who we really are, all the old patterns of behaviour that are no longer helpful, all the fears we have.

For some of us this means rearranging our entire lives so that we become the most important person rather than the least important.

Most of us know we have too much stuff in our lives but we like to hoard things in case we might need them some day.

We hoard physical stuff because we don't think there is enough to go around, but what we are doing is clogging up our lives with junk. Just like any living thing, our physical stuff has energy but all stuff has most energy when it's moving. This means if you aren't using it then it is best to send it out into the universe so that someone else might. Recycle all your old stuff. Give it away, sell it, take it to the charity shops, put it on eBay, but don't leave it sitting in a cupboard just because you think you might need it one day. If you really need it one day then you will find it again, or it will find you, or some variation of it will appear in your life.

We hoard emotional stuff. It's okay to hoard memories in our brains because brains have plenty of capacity, but it's not so good for us to hoard memories of feelings. Feelings need to flow. When we hoard them, and we usually hoard painful feelings, we are not letting them flow. We need to get rid of them. Some of us will need to see counsellors to help us work out good ways to process these memories, or we might begin to process them ourselves in any way that we find helpful. Usually this involves actually feeling the feeling and going with it – we might act it out in ritual or pray about it or meditate upon it. But we need to let this emotional stuff go.

We hang onto old patterns of behaviour because we believe they are helpful or because we don't even realise that is what we are doing.

We hoard friends and acquaintances who may no longer need to be in our lives. We hang onto friendships and partners even when neither person is growing through the relationship. We hold onto our children's lives when we should let them go their own way. We hang onto control of people we say we love.

Finally, we all do too much stuff. We do stuff we don't want to do, things we think we should do but hate to do, and stuff that fills our days so that we don't have time to think or feel about what is really important.

All of us have lives filled with stuff that we don't need anymore, stuff that is hindering our growth. We fill up our lives with stuff because we are terrified that when we strip away all the trappings of a physically based life, there will be nothing left.

If we can begin to let go of our past stuff we start to make room for the new. This is the unknown and it is full of scariness because we have learnt to fear what we cannot control. But we are now learning to trust the process. When the process of our lives lets us know that we need to begin to get rid of stuff that we no longer need, we do so. For most of us, what follows is a time of living empty. Sometimes we live empty for quite a long while. However, we can't live empty until we begin to rid our lives of all its stuff. We clear out all the stuff – physical, emotional and mental – that clutters our life. We let it go and in doing so we begin to live empty.

This emptiness is not nothingness. It is not a black hole full of lurking terrors as many people fear. Each of us knows this emptiness because we live with it every day. We try to fill it with people and things; we try to avoid it by keeping ourselves busy and doing more and more stuff.

We all know these things don't fill the emptiness inside. We cannot eat ourselves full, or drink ourselves full or take drugs to fill this emptiness. Work, relationships, sex, religion – none of these will fill our emptiness. There is only one thing that will fill this emptiness and that is our inner self – our soul and its connection to spirit. Within the emptiness exists our inner self but we have trouble finding it because we are always trying to fill this space with other things.

The challenge is to get rid of the old and live empty for a while. Resist the urge to fill the space with anything except an increasing awareness of self. You gradually learn what it is you need to make your life whole.

Principle 9 – Always be willing to change

Elizabeth Kubler Ross wrote about the five stages of grief involved in death and dying.[26]

4. Denial

5. Anger

6. Bargaining

7. Depression

8. Acceptance

Every time we face a change in our lives, it is similar to what we face when a loved one dies. It is a process of going through the stages until we reach acceptance and move on. As we heal ourselves, some part of us is dying just as another part of us is being reborn. The deaths are really deaths of old beliefs, deaths of our ideas about how the world works, deaths of patterns of behaviour that no longer nurture us. These mini deaths are difficult. We resist them and classically, we resist them in these five stages.

We don't need to go through all the stages in order, or all of them in depth, but it serves us well to remember that in some sense we experience them every time we go through the process of change.

When my marriage and my working life were both foundering, I spent several years in denial. There was nothing wrong. Everything was fine. I was happy and I had everything I wanted.

I look back at this denial stage as one where I was in some sort of trance state. Denial is such an unconscious phase that when we

---

26   On Death and Dying, Elizabeth Kubler Ross.

are in it we have no idea at all. We actually think and believe that everything is okay.

At some point, I realised quite suddenly that there was a problem in the marriage and I entered the anger stage. I first turned my anger on my husband – he didn't understand me, he didn't listen to me. If only he could do this or that, then we wouldn't have a problem. Then I got angry with myself, partly for being in denial for so long! Then I got angry at the world for its expectations.

I then entered bargaining and attempted counselling. If he would try this, then I would do that. We both flipped between anger and bargaining and sometimes tried going back to denial for a while.

Then came the period of depression, which was a seemingly endless time where nothing happened at all and both of us were suffering.

Eventually we worked through the depression to reach some acceptance and we decided to be apart. For a while afterwards we would both flip back to anger, bargaining and depression as we gradually resolved the issues.

This is an oversimplification, because there were other mini deaths happening at the same time and for which the same process occurred. I had to deal with the death of the marriage, the death of the family unit, the death of an imagined life, and many more minor deaths of my ideas about how the world worked. I also had to deal with my daughters going through the same process at different speeds and cycles.

In learning from these mini deaths, we do so by doing the work of depression, as M. Scott Peck would say.[27] Depression in

27   The Road Less Travelled, M. Scott Peck.

this instance is not always the debilitating depression that requires antidepressants and therapy, which is just a more severe form.

Depression is that phase where we feel that there is no answer, where the perceived loss is so large that we have trouble understanding how our lives will ever get back to normal. If we have the idea that we can revert to our old life, then we miss the whole point. Something is dying or has died; things have to change for us to move on. We cannot go back, we can only go forward.

The work of depression is in finding our way forward.

This is the work of healing. We are transforming ourselves into wholeness. It is the practical side of our lessons. It is casting off the parts of ourselves that we are finally ready to let go of. It is the mini deaths that lead us further along our path. It is like peeling off the layers of an onion to discover more about ourselves. It is about shedding those patterns of behaviour that no longer work for us.

All of above nine principles help us deal with chaos more easily. As we bear these in mind, let us look at how we might better deal with chaos on a practical level.

THREE - DEALING WITH CHAOS

Life is full of chaos. When we feel ourselves out of control is when we most need to remember how to be whole. My theory is that chaos is designed to heal fragmentation, to bring the system back to balance and harmony, to bring the system back to wholeness. On an individual level, chaos is what helps us heal. Our fragmentation is healing. We may not be connected to our deeper self, we may not be connected to the rest of the system, we may be out of balance, or the system may be out of balance. Healing ourselves is never just about us as an individual but always also about the larger system. As with all systems, it is immensely complex. There are no simple answers.

How we deal with chaos in our lives is something we have more control over. Chaos may arise as an illness, or it may come in many other guises. However it comes, we can deal with it better if we understand a few basic features of the chaotic process.

1. There is no cause and effect – there is no one thing to blame for our illness or disease.

2. The non-linear process of chaos does not reach an outcome until the process has finished.

3. Because there is no cause and effect, we cannot control the process using linear methods.

4. We do not yet know how to control a non-linear process. It may be that there is no way to control these processes.

5. We can control our own reactions and behaviour. Dealing with chaos means dealing with our reactions and behaviours.

The following steps are part of a cycle that we need to keep paying attention to when we find ourselves in chaos.

1. Awareness

The process that I have called chaos is any process that occurs in our life where we don't feel comfortable or where we feel out of control. This is because in a logical sense, we are out of control. The process of life (chaos) is transforming us (or the system). This process can be a physical illness, an emotional illness, a spiritual crisis, an environmental crisis, or any situation where we feel uncomfortable, out of control or chaotic.

The first step in dealing with chaos is to become aware that this is what is happening. We are in a chaotic process.

Once we become consciously aware of this, we can then take the necessary steps that allow us to follow the process in a healthier way. While we remain unaware and unconscious of being in chaos, we persist in trying less healthy means of gaining some control.

When we feel uncomfortable and out of control, it is because we are. All we need to do to begin to defuse our panic is to become aware that we are in a chaotic process. We cannot control this type of process in logical ways. We cannot use our linear logic to fix things for us. The process needs to occur to reach an outcome. We can't control the outcome, but we can control our response in a chaotic situation.

2. Take a step back

The next step is to take a step back out of the chaos. Remove yourself from your drama for a few moments and remember the critical things about chaos. We remember that we need to trust ourselves and trust the process. We remember that we need to let go of the illusion that we can control the outcomes. We must surrender control to our inner self and spirit. The process will occur and all we need to do is live it. This is the difficult part and the part we are most often stuck in. We don't want to surrender control. Remembering that our inner self and spirit will guide us through the transformation makes it easier.

Taking a step back and removing ourselves from the drama requires that for a time we become very yin. Metaphorically speaking, chaos is usually very yang and destructive so we might become yin in order to see the bigger picture. We become still in the drama of our lives and try to remove ourselves from that drama. Primarily, we need to get out of our left brain, which is frantically thinking of ways to control the process. We take a step back from our thinking self and become more of an observer.

3. Focus on the parts of the whole self – balance

There are three broad parts to focus on when we find ourselves in chaos. The first is that we need to find our balance – we need to centre ourselves. The second is that we need to establish harmony with those around us – we need to stabilise ourselves. The third is that we need to identify and go with the cycles of life – we need to go with the flow. We are centring ourselves, stabilising ourselves and going with the flow all at the same time.

It is like being adrift in a canoe on a raging river. To get to the other side of the rapids we need to balance our self, and we do this best by finding our centre or sitting in the centre of the boat. Here we have the best possible balance. Then we stabilise ourselves. In the river, we might link up with other canoes. In life, we link up with our support system. Then we go with the flow. We steer where we can but we don't attempt to fight against the current. Rather, we go with it in a balanced and stabilised way. First, we must look at our own balance.

The other day I woke up feeling strange. The world seemed not quite right. I tried to sit up and the room started to spin. I lay down again and it kept spinning. I tried moving my head from side to side and the spinning got much worse. I started to feel very sick.

Gradually as I lay very still the spinning stopped. I had to go to the bathroom so I sat up on the edge of the bed. Everything spun again. After five minutes, it had settled enough that I could lurch into the bathroom. I had no balance so I had to grab onto the wall so that I wouldn't fall. I sat down and felt really sick. Eventually the spinning stopped but as soon as I moved, it started up again. I made it back to my bed without vomiting, but only just. As I lay there feeling the world spin around me, I wondered what I had done to get so out of balance. In the past, I'd had similar episodes of classic vertigo, where the balance mechanism in our inner ear is not working. Sometimes it's caused by a virus, sometimes by junk in the semicircular canals.

Whatever had caused it, there was nothing I could do but lie very still. The slightest movement would bring on the spinning and nausea but if I lay very still I had no symptoms. Clearly, my body just wanted me to be still. So I was. I lay completely still for a whole day – something we don't tend to do in our busy lives. It took me another two days to recover. I learnt a lot through the illness. I learnt that I need other people in my life, that I can't always look after myself. I learnt that sometimes I go around in circles and that I need to pay better attention to where I am going and how much I am doing. I learnt that our sense of balance is very important but it's a sense we completely take for granted.

We all know about the five basic senses – vision, taste, hearing, touch, and smell. We have other senses that we don't pay much attention to. Our sense of balance is one that we rarely pay much attention to unless it doesn't work very well. We pay attention when we get motion sickness, or if we drink too much alcohol or when we get vertigo.

Our sense of balance is governed by a small apparatus in our inner ear called the semicircular canals. These very clever little canals are three circular tubes arranged in three planes. The flow of fluid in the canals lets us know where we are in three-dimensional physical space.

We don't pay balance much attention until we don't have it. In the bigger picture, many of our problems are caused by a loss of balance but we don't always realise this.

Many diseases arise from a lack of balance. Remember the sphere (on the front cover) that is the earth. The initial balance we look at is the balance between light and dark or yin and yang.

Yin receives and contracts into our self, yang gives and expands out towards others. Give and take. Breathe in, breathe out. This is the basis of all balance – in and out, give and take.

Energy flows in and out and the way it flows is dictated by yin and yang. Energy flows in through yin and out through yang. Typically, Western society has an excess of yang. We are all focused on doing and acting and we forget that to be balanced we also need to receive energy.

People who are predominantly yang will run themselves ragged because they feel they always need to be busy doing things. People who are predominantly yin will do too little and become sluggish and depressed. We all need the balance. We need to balance our yang activities with our yin activities. Yang activities are active, fast, doing, making, building. Yin activities are reflective, slow, relaxing, recharging.

We get out of balance in four main ways. We give too much, we take too much, we give too little, or we take too little. Of course, there are variations on this. Sometimes we give too much of what no-one needs, or we take too much of things we don't actually need. The essence of balance for an individual is therefore to give what you need to give and receive what you need to receive. If the individual can achieve this, then they play their whole part in the greater system.

This is all part of what we are learning. What do I need to receive to be whole and healthy and happy? What do I need to give?

4. Focus on stability

We need to connect with the rest of the system and therefore stabilise our self. We do this by asking for help and by surrounding ourselves with people and things that help support us. We pay attention to our connections with other people and the ether.

In my work chaos, I had become aware that I was stuck in the middle of a chaotic process. I had taken a step back and begun the process of balancing myself by focusing on all my parts. To focus on stability means to ask for help and guidance, thus my visit to the clairvoyant tarot reader as a first step. He was able to help me begin to tap into my intuition. The next step was to ask for more help because that is how we stabilise ourselves. We tie our canoes together and form a more stable craft in the raging river. I asked my friends for help and I talked to my boss about the stress at work. I tried to come up with ways to change this.

Stabilising ourselves is not about giving up the responsibility of change and healing to other people. It is about using our social networks to support our transformation. We do not rely upon other people to tell us what to do but rather use their wisdom to complement our own.

5. Focus on the problem and its parts

Next, we focus on the problem and its parts. First, we identify the parts of the problem that we have some measure of control over and then we prioritise and plan what we can do.

Second, we identify the parts of the problem we have no control over and surrender control of those parts. We let go of old patterns of behaviour.

Third, we recognise the paradox of surrendering yet still steering where necessary. We go with the flow but we don't chuck away our paddles and throw our arms up in the air. Rather, we steer to avoid obstacles and to keep ourselves going forward. We relax into the process. This is very hard to do because all our instincts scream at us that we have to do something to avoid catastrophe.

In my work, I needed to give up the idea I could control what work I was doing and accept that for the moment I needed to work in my current job. I had signed a contract knowing that I needed to learn something about commitment. I had to commit myself to the job for the next year. I had to let go of the old pattern of behaviour, which was to change jobs whenever I got to this point in my life. I knew this was a new lesson about changing the way I worked and to do this I needed to make a commitment to my current job. My inner guidance told me this.

What parts of the problem did I have some control over? I had a measure of control over how much I was working. Did I need to work fewer hours, or change some of the work I was doing? Doing either of these was tinkering around the edges, but it might help with my balance. The tarot reader had told me to look after myself better out of work, to work, rest and play instead of just working and resting as I had been doing. I needed to do more things out of work that brought me joy and I needed to work on doing that.

6. Plan what to do and then do it – make the changes

Our left brain is useful for planning and prioritising. So we use it. We plan what we can do that will help us in this situation. We take the smallest steps necessary in order to keep our balance. If all we can do seems insignificant compared to the amount of chaos we find ourselves in, we do not despair. We just do what we can to make even a small difference. That small difference might involve getting some of our needs met that we had denied we had. It might involve becoming aware of how we are not being part of the larger system, so we take small steps to balance ourselves, small steps to stabilise ourselves, and small steps to learn how to go with the flow better. These are the three parts we are learning about – balance, stability and going with the flow.

We are also learning that life is about making changes and transforming ourselves and our lives. We must make the necessary changes. We can't just sit back and do nothing. In my work, I had to make some changes. I wasn't yet sure what the changes entailed exactly but I knew that I had to change the way I was working. It would take many small steps but I knew it involved changing my behaviour. I needed to go back to being a more holistic doctor. I had been sucked into the system and I had lost my holistic approach, so I needed to find it again. I wasn't sure how I was going to do it but I knew that was what I needed to work on.

7. Go with the flow

Going with the flow is essentially about learning how to relax into the process of chaos, the process of life. It is about trusting that the process is taking us where we are meant to be going. So we sit back and enjoy the ride. We pay attention to the parts and try to balance them. We pay attention to the larger systems we are part of and go with the flow of life. We stop struggling and fighting and instead relax into our life.

This does not mean that we don't steer, but that we steer with the flow rather than fight against it.

So here I was feeling discontented about a job that I was committed to for another year at the very least. I was not happy with the way I was working but I was finding it very hard to do anything different. I was finding it hard to give up old patterns of behaviour in my work but for the time being, I didn't know what else to do so I went with the flow.

FOUR - HOLISTIC HEALING

Healing is a natural part of who we are. If we cut ourselves, the natural process is for the cut to heal. If we get a cold, our natural immunity works to fight the cold. If we break our leg, it is usual for this to heal itself. With all these situations, there are factors that enhance the healing and factors that decrease the healing, but healing is a natural process.

The best way to remain healthy is not to get sick in the first place. This is prevention. We are all healthier when we live whole lives filled with passion and joy. To do this we try to follow the process of life and pay attention to our inner selves. Illness mainly occurs when we are not paying attention to our inner selves. Illness is the chaos that attempts to bring us back to wholeness.

Illness holds the seed to healing if we are able to pay it attention. Once we are ill we have entered the process of chaos and therefore we can no longer control it. We have to follow the process and in doing so learn more about ourselves and how we are not being whole. Our inner self knows what will heal us so we need to learn how to connect with our inner self in order to heal. It helps if we are aware. This awareness is of the wholeness. It is an awareness of the interconnectedness of everything. It is an awareness of the dimensions beyond the physical. It is the awareness that there is more to this life than we can perceive physically.

We all want simple answers about how to heal ourselves but this isn't how things work. There are no clear-cut answers – we have to find them for ourselves. How do we find them? By following the process of our lives. I know I am going in circles and repeating myself here but this is what happens in all our lives. We go round in circles or spirals until we learn what we have to learn. What we are learning about is how to live whole lives.

Whenever an illness strikes, we need to remind ourselves of the principles of healing and the steps in dealing with chaos. We become aware that it is likely we are in a process of chaos and the outcome, although unpredictable, will likely be growth towards wholeness and a lessening of fragmentation. So we trust ourselves and the process and allow it to occur without battling too much about the unfairness of it.

We seek help in whatever ways feel right for us and of course, this depends upon the problem and its severity. If we have crushing central chest pain and feel as if we are dying, we don't do a rune reading, we just call the ambulance. Many of our problems require medical intervention, but we are still doing the healing. Doctors and other health professionals will work with the natural healing ability of the body in order to bring the body back into balance.

When we get sick, we often have to revisit the basics. What is my body telling me? How am I feeling? What is my logical brain saying? What is my intuition saying? What are the messages from the ether and the people around me? We look at all our parts in order to help us heal. We wait and see what happens. We can't rush healing. No matter how much we want to be better today, we have to wait until the process has its way. This may sometimes take months.

I had upper arm and shoulder pain for some months when writing this book. Nothing seemed to have caused it and nothing seemed to make it better. I saw a doctor who ruled out anything serious but was unable to tell me what was causing it. I saw a friend who is a kinesiologist and she gave me some relief but the pain persisted. Even though I was writing a book about holistic healing, I couldn't heal myself. I was stuck again. The outcome I wanted was for my arms to stop hurting. The outcome my inner self was working towards could have been completely different. I revisited the principles of healing.

Trust myself and the process. Let go of the desire to control the outcome. Pay attention.

Paying attention means paying attention to all my parts and to what is going on around me. So I sat with that for a while. What was my body trying to tell me? I looked up arm pain in a book. I chose Your Body is Telling You to Love Yourself by Lise Bourbeau because it was the first one I found on my bookshelf. It told me that pain in the arms might signify that I no longer felt useful and that I doubted my capacities, or that I had trouble holding someone close to me. Both of these could be true for me so I mulled this over for a while.

I tried to assess whether I was blocking my feelings in some way. As I sat with my feelings, I noticed a feeling of sadness arise. I was sad about several things in my life at the time. I was going through a transition and there was much change. I had left the job I had found so hard and was starting another in a month. I was moving back to Melbourne from Ballarat. I was unable to sell my house in Apollo Bay so I would have to rent in Melbourne. My children had now all finished school. My partner might have been unable to get a job in Melbourne. So much uncertainty and change was around me that it was no wonder I was not sicker!

I tried to make logical sense of it all. My arms were in some way taking on the weight of the world. It might be that until everything settled down in my life, my arms were a way for me to focus upon myself rather than just get on with what needed to be done.

My intuition had been sending me dreams about water and rivers and battling against the current. Obviously, I needed to stop battling so much against life and just go with the flow. I was in the middle of chaos and I didn't know where I would end up. I decided to draw a rune but I couldn't find them in any of my boxes. I did however find some angel cards so I drew one of those. It told me all was well – everything was happening exactly as it was supposed to, with hidden blessings I would soon understand. This was reassuring and really, what I had been writing about all along. Everything that happens to us is in some way engineered by our inner self and spirit.

I stopped agonising over what was going on and just relaxed. My arms lost some of their tension and I felt lighter. The pain didn't disappear but it lessened and I knew I was on the right track.

I reminded myself of the other principles – take responsibility, remember your lessons, let go of the past, and always be willing to change. I decided that as I was moving to Melbourne, it was a good time to go through my physical stuff and to get rid of some of my possessions. I looked at what I might need to change about myself and decided that as I was starting a new job, it was a good chance to change the way I practised and to become more holistic again. I meditated on what old patterns of behaviour I might let go.

I had some more answers but I knew this pain in my arms was not going to go until I had fully resolved what it was trying to tell me. Maybe I would need the pain for a while. One of the things we need to resolve in ourselves is the need to have everything settled right now. We often have to wait and see what will happen. Time must pass before everything becomes clear. I cannot emphasise this too much. It takes time for us to heal our illness. Time, and reflection on the meaning of the illness for us personally.

A week later, I woke in the night after a dream and knew that the pain in my arms was related in some way to not embracing my life. I was being a passive bystander and not embracing everything in my life. I continued to reflect on this and how I might embrace all aspects of my life. The arm pain seemed to lessen but still didn't go away. I still had things to learn.

Some pain and illness is acute and we heal and learn more about ourselves in a short time. Some illness is chronic and stays with us for much of our lives. How do we heal these diseases? Healing is about aligning our inner and outer selves and becoming more whole. Sometimes we need a chronic disease to help us do this. Sometimes we just don't listen well enough unless we have these chronic diseases. I think my friend with diabetes needs the constant reminder of his physicality that the diabetes gives him. Many chronic diseases are present to remind us that we are human in physical bodies. I don't pretend to understand everything about illness but I do know that many chronic diseases can be cured if we are more open to healing ourselves.

Many chronic diseases are lifestyle disorders – we eat the wrong food, don't exercise enough, don't sleep enough, and don't pay attention to what we really need in our lives. These diseases can be healed but sometimes they take major changes that we are not willing to make.

Healing is not so much about getting rid of our illness as about finding out more about the needs of our inner self and trying to meet those needs. This is how we become whole again. Sometimes even when we are whole we still have chronic illness. This is a paradox and to our logical mind, it seems to go against what I have been writing about. However, this is part of holism – not everything has a logical conclusion. That is why this book has been so difficult to end. I keep looking for a logical conclusion to tie up all the loose ends. But there is none. The end of this book doesn't have a final answer but rather it just leads onto more questions about holism and healing. How can we have illness and still be whole? How can we heal our chronic diseases?

Just as there is always more to learn in life, there is always more to learn about holistic healing. This book is just a start. I hope it enables you to learn how to follow the process better. To learn how to dance with life and to begin to live a whole life.

BIBLIOGRAPHY

The following list of books includes those that I have found to be most influential in helping me shape and define my current beliefs. The authors don't claim to have all the answers but they know how to ask very good questions. Like all good books, they challenge the way we think about things.

Auel, Jean M. The Clan of the Cave Bear. Coronet 2002.

Ballentine, Rudolph. Radical Healing. Random House 1999.

Blum, Ralph. The Book of Runes. Angus and Robertson 1993.

Capra, Fritjof. The Tao of Physics: An exploration of the parallels between modern physics and eastern mysticism. Flamingo, Harper Collins 1983.

Capra, Fritjof. The Turning Point. Flamingo, Harper Collins 1982.

Davies, Brenda. Journey of the Soul: Awakening ourselves to the enduring cycle of life. Hodder and Stoughton 2002.

Davies, Paul. The Mind of God: Science and the search for ultimate meaning. Penguin 1992.

Dawkins, Richard. The God Delusion. Bantam Press 2006.

Edwards, Gill. Wild Love. Piatkus 2006.

Fowler, James W. Stages of Faith: The psychology of human development and the quest for meaning. Collins Dove 1987.

Gerber, Richard. Vibrational Medicine for the 21st Century: A complete guide to energy healing and spiritual transformation. Piatkus 2000.

Gleick, James. Chaos: The amazing science of the unpredictable. Vintage 1988.

Green, Brian. The Elegant Universe: Superstrings, hidden dimensions and the quest for the ultimate theory. Vintage 2000.

Hablitzel, William E. Dying was the best thing that ever happened to me: Stories of healing and wisdom along life's journey. Hachette Australia 2007.

Hay, Louise. You Can Heal Your Life. Hay House 1999.

Hillman, James. The Soul's Code: In search of character and calling. Random House 1996.

Hillman, James. The Force of Character, and the lasting life. Random House 1999.

Kaptchuk, Ted J. The Web that has no Weaver: Understanding Chinese Medicine. Contemporary Books 2000.

Krebs, Charles. A Revolutionary Way of Thinking. Hill of Content 1998.

Kubler-Ross, Elizabeth. On Death and Dying. Tavistock Publications 1970.

Levoy, Gregg. Callings: Finding and following the authentic life. Thorsons 1997.

Long, James. Ferney. Harper Collins 1998.

Mehl-Madrona, Lewis. Coyote Medicine. Fireside 1998.

Moore, Thomas. Soul Mates: Honoring the mysteries of love and relationship. Harper Collins 1994.

Moore, Thomas. Dark Nights of the Soul: A guide to finding your way through life's ordeals. Piatkus 2004.

Myss, Caroline. Anatomy of the Spirit. Bantam Books 1997.

Myss, Caroline and Shealy, C. Norman. The Creation of Health. Bantam Books 1999.

Peck, M. Scott. The Road Less Travelled. Random House 1985.

Pinkola Estes, Clarissa. Women Who Run with the Wolves. Rider 1998.

Pollack, Rachel. Seventy-eight Degrees of Wisdom. Thorsons 1997.

Powers, Rhea and Bantle, Gawain. Riding the Dragon: The power of committed relationship. North Star Publications 1995.

Roberts, Jane. Seth Speaks: A Seth Book. Bantam Books 1974.

Roberts, Jane. The Seth Material: A Seth Book. Bantam Books 1970.

Roberts, Jane. The Nature of Personal Reality: A Seth Book. Bantam Books 1980.

Schulz, Mona Lisa. Awakening Intuition: Using your mind-body network for insight and healing. Bantam 1999.

Sheehy, Gail. New Passages: Mapping your life across time. Harper Collins 1995.

Segal, Inna. The Secret Language of Your Body: The essential guide to healing. Blue Angel Gallery 2007.

Simmons, Philip. Learning to Fall: The Blessings of an imperfect Life. Hodder 2002.

Tolle, Eckhart. A New Earth: Awakening to your life's purpose. Penguin 2005.

Villoldo, Alberto. The Four Insights: Wisdom, power and grace of the earthkeepers. Hay House 2006.

Virtue, Doreen. Angel Medicine. Hay House 2004.

Weiss, Brian. Same Soul, Many Bodies. Piatkus 2004.

Williamson, Marianne. Return to Love. Aquarian/Thorsons 1992.

Williamson, Marianne. Enchanted Love: The mystical power of intimate relationships. Simon and Schuster 1999.

Wilson Schaef, Anne. Beyond Therapy, Beyond Science: A new model for healing the whole person. Harper Collins 1992.

Zukav, Gary. The Dancing Wu Li Masters. Harper 2001.

www.ingramcontent.com/pod-product-compliance
Lightning Source LLC
Chambersburg PA
CBHW072100040426
42334CB00041B/1620